The International Library

T0229948

THE FOUNDATIONS OF
COMMON SENSE

Founded by C. K. Ogden

The International Library of Psychology

GENERAL PSYCHOLOGY
In 38 Volumes

THE FOUNDATIONS OF COMMON SENSE

A Psychological Preface to the Problems of Knowledge

NATHAN ISAACS

Foreword by Sir Cyril Burt

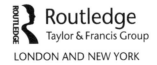

Routledge
Taylor & Francis Group
LONDON AND NEW YORK

First published in 1949 by
Routledge and Kegan Paul Ltd
2 Park Square, Milton Park, Abingdon, Oxfordshire OX14 4RN
711 Third Avenue, New York, NY 10017

First issued in paperback 2014

Routledge is an imprint of the Taylor and Francis Group, an informa business

British Library Cataloguing in Publication Data
A CIP catalogue record for this book
is available from the British Library

The Foundations of Common Sense
ISBN 978-0-415-21027-0
General Psychology: 38 Volumes
ISBN 0415-21129-8
The International Library of Psychology: 204 Volumes
ISBN 0415-19132-7

ISBN 13: 978-1-138-87529-6 (pbk)
ISBN 13: 978-0-415-21027-0 (hbk)

FOREWORD

by Sir Cyril Burt

Mr. Nathan Isaacs is already known for his valuable contributions both to philosophy and (in association with the late Susan Isaacs) to child psychology. He himself needs no introduction ; but I should like to emphasise that, while his book is a profound and valuable contribution to philosophy, it is at the same time based upon a sound psychology. Since modern psychology is a young and rapidly changing science, even the ablest of contemporary philosophers is apt to lapse into a naive or out-of-date type of psychology when he comes to deal with problems of mind or knowledge.

In his new book, Mr. Isaacs seeks to explain how we come to believe in our common sense world, and why, in spite of all philosophical criticism, we cannot help still believing in it. His aim is to show how we progressively build up the various constituents of that belief, and how those constituents tend to support and reinforce one another in a single, well-consolidated structure.

Such an account must consist, not in a reasoned or deductive system of epistemological principles or of metaphysical conclusions. It is essentially a matter of describing, in accurate psychological language, our own states and experiences so far as they can be observed, and in particular the structural pattern which those states and experiences impose upon our tacit assumptions and habitual perceptions. Here Mr. Isaacs brings the latest contributions of psychological understanding to bear upon time-honoured problems of philosophy.

He argues that a complete account of our experience—genetic, historical, and dynamic—must come before any attempt at philosophic argument or criticism. Otherwise the latter will have to work on unstable ideas or fragmentary data, and its results must therefore of necessity collapse as soon as they are examined. Hitherto philosophers have claimed the central issues of knowledge as their own special preserve ; and psychologists, by accepting this claim, have unwittingly helped to maintain the sterile position thus adopted. But a bold and comprehensive psychological description of the whole phenomena in question can contribute something which neither the epistemologist nor the metaphysician can possibly ignore.

Mr. Isaacs' essay should therefore be of the greatest interest and value to students of philosophy and psychology alike, and to those members of the general public who may have felt shaken or disturbed by the current philosophic criticisms of our common notions of truth and reality as we use them in ordinary everyday life.

TABLE OF CONTENTS

INTRODUCTION

The following essay claims no inherent novelty. But its argument is being newly presented because it has so far been largely unheeded and because I think that at present it can be stated more directly, more comprehensively, and (as I hope) more convincingly than was possible in the past.

Put most baldly and summarily, my central thesis is that an adequate empirical account of knowledge must precede any philosophic discussion of its problems. The first stress falls here on "adequate"; and "precede" should be given its full weight, negatively as well as positively. (There is no suggestion of *super-session*.) "Must" means : if philosophic discussion is to avoid *gratuitous* shortcomings, confusions, deadlock and sterility. An "adequate" empirical account of knowledge signifies a systematic description of the relevant psychological facts, based on direct empirical study in their actual psychological context, and in their relations, connections and interdependences with the rest of that context. What this implies in the concrete will, I trust, emerge fully as the argument proceeds.

It should be added that the present essay is a greatly abridged re-statement of a two-volume study completed in 1939 (under the title of *The Theory and Practice of Knowledge*), but still awaiting an opportunity of publication. It is thus no more than an outline sketch, which must perforce leave a vast deal unsaid. Moreover it will be necessary to plunge straight into the middle of our theme, without the preliminary building up which my fuller study provided for and which seemed to me required to bring out the real significance of the enterprise. I believe that it has quite a strong claim to the interest of the thinking general reader, as well as of psychologists and philosophers. But without a great deal of prefatory apparatus there is a risk that the former, and indeed even psychologists, may see little point in an elaborate attempt to establish positions which they consider it best just to take for granted. It may well seem as if the present thesis is entirely a matter between the writer and the philosophers whom, apparently, he is addressing ; it is for them to accept or reject, reply to or disregard the argument, according to their views on its merits. Neither the psychologist nor the general reader without any special interest in philosophy may feel greatly concerned.

However, all this is, I believe, a profound mistake. It may be useful, therefore, to adumbrate in this introduction at least the broad plan of the first volume of the larger work, to serve as a framework for the detailed argument to follow.

What the reader is invited to visualise is a large dramatic picture on the great historic canvas of the emergence and growth of our empirical sciences during the last three hundred years. The main pattern is very familiar : one after another of these sciences has broken away from the original matrix of philosophy, pursued its own autonomous course under the distinctive ægis of the methods of empirical investigation, experiment and test, and flourished exceedingly. And last of all, psychology, with much difficulty but at length triumphantly, has followed suit and become in our day a fully-fledged natural science, young but vigorously thrusting forward and growing, like the rest.

But the part of the picture to which I wish to draw attention is this : in order to be able to break away, psychology has had to leave behind, as inalienably belonging to philosophy, what is in fact a central portion of its own domain. That has been the price paid for its freedom. The matters with which the philosophic theory of knowledge is concerned : the nature of knowledge, its elemental data, the theory of truth, the question of the existence of an objective world and how we can know about this, the basis and the validity of the notion of causality, etc.—all these are equally fundamental for an adequate psychology of cognition, and through this for an adequate science of our psychic life as a whole. If we cannot build up any ordered and stable and comprehensive science about them, our psychology cannot make coherent sense at all. Right at its centre there is a quicksand instead of firm ground, and in order to be " scientific " it is impelled, as it were, to run away from itself. Thus it tends to become superficial and peripheral, largely physiological, or narrowly behaviouristic, and crudely imitative of the other recognised natural sciences where, according to the true scientific spirit and in proper adaptation to its subject-matter, it should establish its own distinct pattern.

This of course is greatly condensed and telescoped and cannot be fully developed here ; also there are important qualifications which will be referred to in their appropriate place. What chiefly concerns us, for our introductory purpose, is to set the following main features and consequences of our picture in the right relief.

(1) It can easily be shown that in the nature of the process of emergence of " scientific " psychology from its philosophic matrix, a vast historic vicious circle has been set up, which now automatically renews itself, and is almost impossible to break through. (The natural attitude of non-interest of psychologists, as well as most general readers, to a critique of the psychology of philosophers might itself be viewed as one manifestation of this state of affairs.) But if the circle is once seen and understood, in all its far-flung workings, the battle is won, because it *can* then be broken.

(2) In the simplest form of that circle : because the so-called philosophic problems of knowledge seem to represent, on all their historical record, the most perplexing and incurable mysteries of human thought, they are regarded as just the kind of ultimate question which philosophy is " there for." And it seems self-evident that psychology, if it is to be as other positive sciences and to prosper, must studiously keep away from them. But just because the positive science within whose field they belong keeps away from them, they maintain their past record and remain in the characteristic state of a hopeless philosophic morass.— That is our thesis, which can, however, itself only be made good by boldly invading the traditional preserves of philosophic epistemology and *demonstrating* how much they have to offer to a strictly empirical-psychological approach (though this must of course be an adequate one).

(3) In effect, it is part of the same circle that we fail to appreciate that in leaving any domain, or any specific problems, to philosophy, what we have really done in the past has been to leave them to the traditional philosophic *method of thought*. And this is one which by its inherent shortcomings and defects must turn into confusion and anarchy whatever it is applied to. With only limited recent qualifications, it is essentially a method of circular dialectical argument and debate, based on the manipulation of mere ideas (usually vague and unstable and equivocal ones), and with the fatal flaw of lack of any preliminary psycholinguistic technique for determining word-meanings.

By way of antithesis, to claim any domain or any problems for empirical science means, in parallel fashion, nothing more than claim them for the empirical scientific method of inquiry. Our accumulated bodies of knowledge called sciences are merely the product of the cumulative application of that particular method. And this is no limited local mystery, but—as our adequate psychology of knowledge, once we have it, brings out—

simply the integration of all we have learnt from our experience about the ways in which we can remedy ignorance and error, applicable in every domain of our experience in which we *wish* to overcome ignorance and to minimise error. (It may well be that in some directions shorter cuts than the full apparatus of observation, experiment and empirical tests are open to us, but if so, the test is that they do in fact lead to cumulative dependable knowledge, not to self-repeating circles of conflict, error and ignorance.) All this will be further developed in our main text, and is only fore-shadowed here for the sake of an advance whole view.

(4) We shall thus try to show that the approach which we call scientific can and must be applied (in the suitable form of a psychology which is contextual and causal, genetic and historical) to the main traditional mysteries of knowing itself. There is no least suggestion indeed that by this approach they can once and for all be solved. Ultimate unsolved mysteries will be left in this field as in every other. But no more, just as no less. We have open to us exactly the same possibility of building up a body of organised positive knowledge or science about all the central facts of knowledge as about each part or aspect of the physical world and every other part of the psychological world. The mystery need only come at the end instead of preventing us from ever making a beginning.

(5) And such a body of knowledge about knowing is of vital importance not only to psychology, and so to psychologists, but for very much the same reasons to *every* intelligent and thoughtful person. The themes that are at present left to the philosophic theory of knowledge, and thus to the traditional philosophic assumptions and methods, are the most pivotal and central for *all* our thinking, our social sciences, our education, even the theory of our physical sciences, and our general perspective and outlook. Confusion and instability in this field, and an endless battle of rival ambiguous and shifting views, mean a deep underlying confusion, instability and incapacity for resolving differences or achieving agreement throughout all those realms of social thought where systematic empirical science has gained no firm purchase yet—and is in fact held at bay precisely by these conditions. Yet the ordinary intelligent person soon ceases even to try to get to the root of such matters, because he in turn knows, or thinks he knows, that they belong within the realm of the most hopeless philosophic snares and mysteries. A little experience rapidly convinces him that it is useless to let himself get caught in them ;

he can get no further, and sooner or later he has no choice, if he wants to get back to any of his more positive interests and pursuits, but to break away and to keep away.

If, however, there is once a positive body of information about such matters as the elements and principles of growth of knowledge, the basic criteria of truth and falsity, the grounds for our belief in an objective reality, the nature of the distinction between fantasy and fact, or the authentic constituents of and evidence for such a master-concept as that of causality, what could be of greater interest and importance to every intelligent and thinking person? These are the most fundamental and pervasive facts and ideas on which our world is built, the basic notions and tools on which our lives turn every day, and the central supports for all our feelings and actions, thoughts and beliefs and even visions.

The present essay cannot follow out in any detail these wider implications of its theme. It can in fact only touch lightly even on that keystone of the arch of our knowledge, the notion of explanation. The consequences for our psychology at large, for our social thinking generally, and for the theory and practice of education will not be drawn here, since they would require further volumes. It should also be emphasised again that this essay does not pretend to go beyond an elementary sketch ; there is a vast deal more material already available, and immense scope for further detailed investigation, in the actual field of the cognitive development of young children. But it is hoped that enough has been said to make out a case for the intrinsic interest and significance of what follows—in the last resort even more from the point of view of the psychologist and the general reader than from that of the traditional philosopher. From the latter's angle this study may only appear as yet another essay in subversion. His business, if he deems it worth attending to at all, is no doubt to seek to convict it of the usual round of philosophic fallacies ; and thus to try to show once more how triumphantly the philosophic circle, and the philosophic jungle, always prevails in the end. But even from his angle I trust that it may seem that there is at least a case to be met. As regards the modern Logical Analysts and still more the Logical Positivists, it will, I hope, be plain that at bottom we are on the same side. I am not really arguing more than that, if our common object is to be achieved, it is necessary to take one more step (even if it is a somewhat radical one) along our common road.

CHAPTER I

INADEQUATE PSYCHOLOGICAL DATA OF THE CURRENT PHILOSOPHIC THEORY OF KNOWLEDGE

(1) We must begin with the fundamental proposition that adequate data for any sort of philosophic theory of knowledge can only be provided by an adequate general picture of our cognitive experience, set in its right place in the context and course of our total experience.

Now current philosophy, in continuing its traditional discussions, takes over most of its psychological data, i.e. the notions, assumptions and examples with which it works, from the past history of these discussions. And they represent only an extremely narrow and very defective selection from our actual experiential material. This selection has in fact never been radically revised and gets little opportunity of revision, just because all the time-honoured controversies are still going on and every one of these notions, assumptions and examples remains caught up in the same secular tangle of arguments which endlessly renews itself. It does so because we never manage to separate arguments about words from arguments about ideas, and arguments about ideas from arguments about facts, and this in turn is largely due to the vagueness, instability and inadequacies of the notions with which we are trying to work, in one great vicious circle.

(2) These last characteristics have been abundantly demonstrated, from a purely logical angle, by the penetrating critical work of the Cambridge Logical Analysts (and to a large extent also by the Vienna school of Logical Positivists). But these critics have only been successful in diagnosing, not in remedying, because they themselves share in the assumption that the *empirical material* (i.e. the actual psychological or phenomenological data) utilised by traditional philosophic thought is all that is needed. Therefore they assume that what is required, in the place of the traditional ways of working with these muddled and shifting notions, is merely to persevere with the task of critical analysis till a set of univocal, clear, precise and stable ideas is built up.

(3) The general history of our knowledge suggests, however, that such ideas can usually only be formed *pari passu* with the building up of connected fabrics of detailed empirical

knowledge, and can neither be fashioned nor sustained in a vacuum, i.e., in the absence of such a fabric. The only apparent exception is that of mathematical concepts ; but there are many grounds for considering them a special case, which we can only assume valid in other fields at our peril. The peril is most strikingly illustrated just by the history of philosophy, and even by the comparative barrenness of its recent Cambridge chapter, which seemed to promise so radical and fruitful a new start. But unfortunately the Cambridge analysts, as well as other philosophers, have debarred themselves from recognising the inadequacy of the psychological material with which they are working through their attitude to the so-called psychological fallacy. Against the claim of some nineteenth century champions of psychology that the theory of knowledge is nothing but a branch of this science, or at the best largely dependent upon it, there has been a vigorous philosophic reaction. It has been insisted that both the philosophic problems of knowledge and the right methods of dealing with them are completely independent of the empirical science of psychology. Furthermore, that the philosophic approach is logically prior, because the empirical science, in common with others, makes various epistemological assumptions, the validity of which it is the business of philosophy to scrutinise and appraise. It must be added that psychologists themselves have tended more and more not only to accept this sharp severance but to underline it on their own account, in order to keep their science free from philosophic entanglements and to assimilate it as much as possible to the most successful of the other natural sciences.

(4) Thus philosophers have more or less deliberately shut themselves within the circle of their own traditional notions, assumptions and selected instances, and have gone on with debates only too capable, on those premises, of renewing themselves in the same form and terms for ever. Nor have most empirical psychologists had much to contribute towards a more satisfactory psychological basis for philosophic thought about knowledge. On the one hand they have tended, for the above reasons, to leave the central regions of knowledge most carefully alone, to the great detriment of their own science, thus deprived of a most crucial portion of its proper subject matter, without which the rest could not make sense. On the other hand, by way of carrying the same warping process still further, empirical psychologists have sought to make their science as good an experimental and laboratory science as the rest, by shifting its focus towards

the periphery of its true field, where alone those techniques could readily be practised.

However, in the past few decades various trends making for a more autonomous and integral psychological approach have asserted themselves : in particular, Gestalt Psychology, in the field of perception and intellectual insight ; Child Psychology, in its focus on the whole individual, and its genetic and historical study of his total development ; and Psycho-Analysis in its purely psychological, yet thoroughly dynamic and causal view of human affective history and behaviour. The tendency to keep away from the supposed special domain of the philosophic theory of knowledge has indeed gone on, and has maintained its unfortunate distorting effects on the progress of the rest of psychology towards full integration. But there have been at least two major exceptions to that tendency. First and foremost there was J. M. Baldwin's *Genetic Logic*, which is a superb survey, from a strictly psychological angle, of the whole genetic deployment of knowledge, and which has shown its practical fertility in the great series of empirical investigations in the same genetic field associated with Professor Piaget. Secondly, a consistent and most penetrating psychological approach to the domain of knowledge has likewise been carried through with invaluable results (not only in the realm of theory but also in that of concrete application to the processes of education) by Professor Dewey. The writer believes that even Baldwin and Dewey are still caught up to some extent in the consequences of the defective empirical psychology which is so deeply entrenched in the entire history of the philosophic theory of knowledge ; and that this face explains not only the stubborn controversies between them, but also certain flaws in the empirical work of their schools. But by a still more radical empirical-psychological approach over the ground won by both, combined with the contributions referred to earlier, it should be possible now to confront that defective psychology with the outline of something far less inadequate and error-riddled, which ought clearly to displace it.

According to a kind of inverse Gresham's Law, by which sooner or later fuller and truer information tends to drive out more fragmentary and erroneous, the greatest part of the physics and chemistry of the Greeks, Scholastics and earlier modern philosophers has long since disappeared from circulation, and no philosophic thinker would now dream of trying to reason in terms of most of their notions and assumptions. The argument here is that the time has come when the same inverse Gresham's Law can begin to be applied to the anachronistic cognitive psychology still so implicitly and unthinkingly used among philosophers.

(5) It is plain that the foregoing thesis challenges trial by actual results, rather than by any mere endeavour to meet the fashionable anti-psychological arguments of philosophers on their own ground. However, to counter strongly-established prejudices, it may be useful to develop a little further the lines on which, as has already been indicated, even the formal anti-psychological case can, on the present view, be met.

(i) The notions and assumptions inherited by current epistemology are just as much empirical psychology (of a sort) as what it is proposed to put in their place. The only difference is that they are archaic, crude and hopelessly defective, and for that very reason give rise to very many of the difficulties in which philosophers become involved and which then, in a vicious circle, cause them to believe that these are elemental mysteries beyond the reach of any mere empirical science. The way in which the process operates can easily be worked out. Philosophy begins in every field with the picking up, from current experience and current language, thought and tradition, of a number of ideas and situations which specially stimulate or provoke reflection and debate. The nature and meaning of these are then considered and discussed, opposing views are developed, and at the same time, since at the outset ideas are naturally vague, words are ambiguous and knowledge is incomplete, every sort of argument arises about what it is that is *really at issue*, which of many competing alternatives represents its true character and essence, how far this supports or necessitates the original views advanced, etc., etc. And when this kind of interaction between reflection, debate, ratiocination, prior beliefs and speculation gets to work on such common floating notions as sensations and ideas, knowledge and truth, reality and appearance, objectivity, causality, etc. ; when it finds itself caught moreover in their interlocking relations and becomes duly confused between word-meanings, ideas and facts, essences and views, there is always so much more to be said, so much to be criticised, so much to be proved, disproved and re-proved, that the process cannot help but go on and on of its own momentum. And inevitably therefore it keeps more or less within its established circle of notions and assumptions without either occasion for or thought of any radical breaking out. (Apparent revolutions like the Kantian and the Hegelian have duly been shown to have introduced no essentially new ideas, nothing which was not already implicit as long ago as Plato. The whole history of philosophy has been one long case of "*plus ça change, plus c'est la même chose,*" and even Aristotle and Aquinas have had their recent revivals. The more recent revolutions, like that of the Logical Analysts, do not even claim to have introduced any new ideas, but on the contrary *emphasise* their merely Augean-stable-cleaning concentration on the old.)

But there is nothing in this self-repeating circle to suggest that the initial stock-in-trade of notions and assumptions represented all or most of the data-material actually available, to say nothing of the further detailed and systematic knowledge *of the same kind* which sustained factual inquiry might have secured. On the contrary even the initial data-material was never properly examined, or re-examined, in its own field, since its very existence, character and status were under continuous dialectical dispute. And the philosophic stock-in-trade did not become any less faulty and incomplete when—over and above the automatic operation of the philosophic cycle—it was deliberately sealed off from its source-field and from all further work on this ; that is to say when, with the full consent of psychologists themselves, this whole realm of ideas and problems was marked out as peculiarly a philosophic preserve and in any case as something logically prior to any mere data-field, or any work on the latter. There were other factors, which will emerge later, to reinforce the sealing-off process. In any case the upshot was that a particular narrow set of empirical ideas and assumptions, representing a first very crude selection from the most obvious portions of an ill-observed and largely unexplored order of facts, was isolated from all the rest and endowed with a quite fictitious status which it naturally could not sustain. For in truth this set of ideas and assumptions is not in the least *different* in kind from an adequate description of the same data-field, but only grossly and devastatingly inferior, within the *same* kind.

(ii) The more adequate description proposed here does *not* require any special epistemological assumptions, which philosophy must first scrutinise and appraise. Indeed from the foregoing argument it follows that if any such assumptions were implicit in an adequate description (i.e. one that is more complete and less riddled with plain empirical errors), they would be at least equally present in the current inadequate one, on which our philosophising itself is based. In fact, of course, philosophers are constantly discovering or uncovering such assumptions in one another : that is part of the self-perpetuating philosophic circle. But the truth is that it is the very advantage of an adequate account that it is far less dependent on any assumed elements than an inadequate version. That is how the latter deals with its gaps and its errors. An adequate description of our experience provides its own homogeneity, coherence and comprehensiveness.

We shall not, in what follows, make more than the barest minimum assumption of even the most subjectivist or solipsistic philosophers : nothing going beyond the experiencing of our own states, or if anyone wishes, my own states. We shall merely aim at something like the picture of their full content, their full range and their actual (historical) order, with every particular kind of state viewed as it concretely occurs within that context, in contrast with the traditional small group of abstracted philosophic fragments.

It may be said that such an account, whatever it may or may not be, cannot pretend to represent the current empirical science of psychology. The latter, just in so far as it has become an authentic science, assumes the ordinary physical world of common sense and science, assumes the ordinary scientific notion of causality, assumes the validity of the principle of induction and of ordinary scientific experimental methods, etc., etc. Our reply, as we have already seen, is in part a critique of much current empirical psychology, supported by a great deal that has been happening in its own field ; in part a critique of many current philosophic assumptions about empirical science, on the ground that even physics and chemistry can be stated perfectly well (if one wishes to trouble) in direct terms of certain ranges of our experiences and our experienced distinctions between them, without the need of any supporting assumptions, whether ontological or methodological. But in the main the picture to be offered must be left to speak for itself. For it will appear precisely that an *adequate* description of our experience as we actually experience it, complete with the experienced distinctions and relations which successively appear within it, maintain themselves in it and form a progressive system of classification and organisation of our further experiences, finishes up by validating in the most decisive way all those assumptions of our ordinary physical world, causality, induction, etc., which all sciences are said to take so much for granted, but which philosophers put so severely on trial. Our ordinary language based on these supposed *assumptions* is merely the simplest and most compact way of summing up an immense number of convergent and inter-supporting experience-constellations, and of registering the cumulative outcome of our whole experience-history. There is no reason accordingly why, in the end, we should not profit by all the advantages of our ordinary language, so long as we are clear that it can always be translated back into the cumulative experience-system it represents.[1] That exactly will be our object here. But thus in turn our purely experiential or phenomenological psychology will prove to be equivalent to the most materialistic or behaviouristic scientific empirical psychology, *provided the latter in turn is adequate.* (That is obviously *not* the case as regards Watsonian behaviourism, or most of our current physiological or laboratory psychology ; but these are already largely surpassed.)

(iii) Finally, it must again be underlined that the present argument in no wise claims that an adequate psychological account of our cognitive experience can take the place of the philosophic consideration of knowledge, or render this superfluous. This essay does not profess to be more than a psychological prelude to the latter, or at any rate to philosophy as a whole. I differ from the Logical Positivists in not thinking even metaphysical questions meaningless ; my criticism would rather be that they suffer from a plethora of meanings, all tangled up with one another and all of them both vague and fluctuating. The remedy for this, however, is not primarily logical or even linguistic analysis, but the provision of a connected context of detailed information in which every idea can be adequately specified and demarcated from every other, and each is, as it were, held in place both by its own concrete content and by that of all the others.

That applies equally to epistemological issues. The detailed context of an adequate description of our cognitive experience merely provides an authentic, stable and orderly subject-matter for our ultimate philosophic problems. No doubt much of the present confusion of verbal, conceptual and real questions will disappear, and the whole procedure of traditional philosophic

---

[1] This may appear to come quite close to the Logical Positivists' distinction and relation between " sense-data " language and " object " language. I have no wish to exaggerate the differences between us, since I am in fact in sympathy with much of their viewpoint. But there are marked differences, which will emerge, and I cannot think their psychology adequate. At best I can only regard it as a sort of two-dimensional projection of a three-dimensional psychological reality—plus an unfortunate tendency to deny or disregard much of the content of the latter. Anyway, if in the light of the later sections of this essay, we are after all in large agreement, so much the better.

thinking, and much even of the more recent logico-analytic approach, may have to be overhauled. But no phenomenological description of our experience, however complete, can relieve us of the desire (whether satisfiable or not) for some sort of total interpretation. Nor can it save us from many loose ends and residual problems, to provide us with concrete grounds for philosophic restlessness and questioning, and in particular, to leave open all sorts of possibilities of *alternative* readings, thought of or still unthought of.

In our concluding section the theme of the place left on our view for philosophy in general and for the philosophic consideration of knowledge in particular will be further reviewed. The main point here is that to say that philosophy must *start* in every field from adequate and accurate phenomenological data rather than from fragmentary and grossly inaccurate ones, is not in the least to put these data in the place of philosophy itself. It constitutes on the contrary the clearest acknowledgment that philosophic thought only begins where the phenomenological description ends.

CHAPTER II

CHIEF FLAWS OF THE TRADITIONAL "PHILOSOPHIC" APPROACH. GENERAL FEATURES OF AN ADEQUATE PSYCHOLOGY OF KNOWLEDGE

(1) At this stage we shall only briefly set out, for purposes of contrast, the main heads of a psychological critique of philosophers' psychology; later sections must provide the concrete detail.

(i) Philosophic discussion still too often deals in notions such as that of " *the* knower," " *the* mind," " *the* subject," " *the* object," etc. These are assumed ideal or essential entities which simply do not exist, and the employment of such notions merely blurs our responsibility for truth or error in relation to any genuine classes of concrete existents. For an adequate empirical psychology there is no such thing as " the knower," but a range of variable knowing individuals, that is, individuals whose experiences and activities yield, *inter alia*, knowledge. In ultimate solipsistic terms I start with only one such individual—but my own experience eventually obliges me to acknowledge a host of others parallel to myself (that is, I have had a multitude of experiences which I have had to summate in that way, and the continuing course of my experiences compels me to maintain this mode of summation).

The notion of " the mind " is a very complicated affair, the correct substitute for which we need not stay to consider here ; but as currently used, it is the negation of precise thinking, and we shall find that we can manage remarkably well without it.

Similarly, there linger on in philosophic literature fictitious mental faculties of a kind which practically all psychologists have long since discarded. Not a few philosophers still talk of " Sense," " Reason," " Thought," etc., virtually as if these were entities in their own right, when all they mean is certain distinguishable ways of experiencing and behaving of certain classes of organic individuals.

(ii) Philosophic discussion works to a large extent with vague, questionable and in some instances invalid data. These include such key-notions as those of " sensations " (or sense-data, or sense-impressions, or sensa), " ideas," " propositions " and " judgments." Though all of them are centres of controversy, they are mostly assumed to correspond to something given, however much debate there may be about what precisely this is in each case. But what is in fact psychologically given is very different from what these abstract-atomic notions suggest. " Sensations " in particular have no claim whatever to be the primary *psychological* units ; the true basic experiential datum is a focalised field. And what is given in the type of experience which philosophers have tended to treat as made up of " sensations " (or " sense-data," etc.) is a focalised *perceptual* field. Similarly " ideas " are not, as is so readily assumed, the universal *given* units of thought. Where they are present, they represent the *last stage reached* in a process, which most often is not carried so far. Where it is not, what we treat as unitary given " ideas " are often the vaguest and most shifting word-centred composites or blurs ; and a vast amount of decomposing, specifying, stabilising and reorganising work has to be done before any really usable units of thought, or true " ideas," can be achieved. —" Propositions " again embrace a most heterogeneous series of psychic contents. Whilst the distinction of the propositional *content* from judgmental or other *attitudes* towards it is right and important, the crucial fact is that the former is as psychological as the latter. Propositions are in effect, primarily, *imagined* or *pictured* or *thought* states of affairs, built up in the first place on the model of representations of a subject (subject-matter, or object, or entity, or occurrence, of any kind), plus some sort of determinate representation *about* this. But that basic pattern then undergoes so many different elaborations and transformations that although all the stages are continuous *inter se*, we cannot hope to understand the true (psychological) significance of the later forms, except by reinstating each of them in its proper place within its right derivation-series.

(iii) The foregoing may be generalised into a broad criticism of the habitual philosophic severance of our real psychological data from their context and connections. We stultify the living elements of our thought if we break them up into separate, isolated, apparently self-contained and self-given units, such as " sense-data ", " ideas ", etc. We cannot begin to *understand* what we are talking about until we have restored each of these pretended units to its proper psychological context, both cross-sectional and timewise, and re-defined it in terms of that, i.e. as both a product and a functional part of it. This will be further illustrated below.

(iv) The traditional philosophic theory of knowledge attends only to a narrow selection of fragments of our total psychic life, and leaves out essential ranges of facts and key-characters even of our cognitive life. This is clearly of outstanding importance. The crucial omissions are (*a*) virtually the whole *psychological* category of action, and (*b*) those most significant *general* features of all our experience—its pervasive *temporal* and *historical* character.

(*a*) Action is not indeed merely omitted. It is treated as obviously a bodily category and thrust into an outer limbo ; i.e. that of the world of the body and other objects, and of externality at large, which the philosophic theory of knowledge has yet to examine for its credentials. The psychology assumed by philosophers only recognises as " mental " certain conventional types of content of our own " states," usually classified as thought, feeling and will, or cognition, affection and volition. These form the common ground of our traditional philosophy and our older academic psychology. Beyond this, our more recent psychology plunges into the outer world. Our philosophic theory of knowledge, on the other hand, selects for its special province an even narrower field, viz., the conventional main members (sense-impressions, doubtfully ; ideas ; judgments and their variants) of the one domain of cognition.

But it is only our established philosophic prejudices which prevent us from seeing that the foregoing sort of psychology is quite wrong. If we are really to carry through the attempt to draw a complete picture of our experience as *experience*, we cannot on any account leave action out. Whatever else it may or may not be, or claim to be, it is certainly a most distinctive and pervasive *mode of experience*. The more sceptical or searching we are about any further claims, the more plainly we are driven to acknowledge at least the phenomenological or psychological characters of the *mode of experiencing* we call that of action. It is quite different in its experienced quality from willing, as well as from desiring or feeling or cognising ; and we find that it has its own regular relations to these other modes, and its own distinctive antecedents and consequences in the cognitive mode. We shall observe, in effect, in any complete account which we seek to give of our experience as we concretely experience it, in its connections and interdependences, that the mode we call action provides the most ubiquitous connecting tissue, and plays the most determining and controlling part. And if we try leaving it out, the whole fabric breaks up into disconnected and incoherent fragments—just such as we do find in the traditional philosophic theory of knowledge. We then naturally cannot make sense of those fragments, and nothing will enable us to do so but the re-instatement of the omitted connecting tissue, and thus the re-integration of our experience as it actually happens. We shall see indeed that the *experiential mode* we call " action " is a particularly vital key to the development of knowledge, in all its distinctive features.[1]

(*b*) Similarly with the temporal and historical character of our experience, which indeed is almost the same thing as saying, the whole character of our experience as experience. What we know, ultimately, is our own cumulative experience-history. We are only aware of " sensations ", " ideas ", " feelings " and all our other psychological and epistemological categories as parts or fragments—living parts or severed fragments—of our experience-history. Our philosophic theory of knowledge takes these elements (or " data ") out of their historical context, and debates and analyses them as static entities. But that again cuts out practically all their meaning, and all our keys to this. If we turn back to our experience itself as we experience it, we must note the direct *temporal* quality of so much of it : memory, expectation, desires, interests, aims, purposes, etc. ; the *timewise flow* of all of it ; the *historical cumulativeness* of its whole course. We shall find indeed that the temporal character of our experience provides the first and most solid and enduring basis for the very notions of knowledge, truth and fact, and for their main validating tests. But our traditional theory of knowledge has to all intents and purposes missed all this. In so far as it considers time at all, it does so only in the form of the timeless, abstract " idea " of time, which then gets dealt with like any other abstracted psychological fragment ; and indeed is in the main left to psychologists as a theme for them.

(v) The traditional philosophic theory of knowledge completely lacks either an empirical-psychological preface to language, or any consciousness of the need for this. Yet nothing is more obviously necessary. Between ourselves and all logical or rational communication with others, there is the screen of language ; it is patently something empirical and psychological, something about which we need to know a great deal and about which we can only learn by empirical-psychological inquiry. And even when we are just thinking for ourselves, or operating within our

---

[1] For our broad purpose here we may include under the notion of action, or active behaviour or experience, that of movement and locomotion, although of course it is in turn a very distinctive and important sub-mode.

own minds, we are (*a*) plainly using our linguistic instrument all the time and depending on it (*b*) plunged into a very late stage of a long empirical-psychological history—all the history by which we ourselves progressively learn to understand and use our language, by which we pick up its implicit assumptions and patterns of thought, and by which we habitually come to treat it, in our familiar way, as something hardly to be distinguished from our thought itself. This history again is something we cannot hope to grasp and appreciate, in all its implications and consequences, except by objective empirical-psychological study.

The results of the lack of any such study, or of any sense of the need for it, constitute what is probably the worst stumbling-block for all our philosophic thinking and discussion. It is clear that so long as we cannot avoid sliding backward and forward between questions of word-meanings, questions of concept-definitions and questions of substance or fact (actualities or realities), in the way we have already described, we have little hope of ever settling or resolving anything. Yet this sliding process seems inevitable so long as we have no recognised technique, resting on established empirical-psychological knowledge, for separating issues of word-meanings from all else and *dealing with them first*. No one is unaware, of course, of the existence of these questions and of the fatal pitfalls which ambiguous, vague and shifting word-meanings can place in the way of valid and effectual thought. But we have only the traditional logico-philosophic remedy of *definition*, the theory of which is itself controversial and which, in the case of all the key-terms involved in past philosophic argument, soon gets drawn into the self-same circle of dispute wherein differences about word-meanings and differences of view about the realities (or supposed realities) referred to can never be pulled apart. A proper empirical-psychological approach to language, entailing, as we have seen, also a genetic and historical one, would automatically lead to the elementary technique needed for isolating and determining the object, or subject-matter, any one of us is talking or thinking *about*, as distinct from and prior to all *views about* this. That technique indeed causes us little difficulty outside the knots into which we have tied ourselves in the philosophic field. But its successful practice, given these knots, also requires proper standards or criteria of the minimum conditions for any viable word-meaning as such.—However, this general theme cannot be further developed here and is not essential to us, since for the terms which chiefly concern us, i.e., those central to the philosophic theory of knowledge, our main approach will furnish meanings sufficiently concrete and massive and organised to be fully self-sustaining.

(2) The foregoing criticisms point to the broad characteristics of the positive empirical psychology of knowledge envisaged here. By way of drawing the threads together we may say, very summarily, that :

(i) it must form an integral part of a comprehensive psychology of human mental life and behaviour
(ii) the subject-matter of such a psychology consists of individual human experience-histories
(iii) its aim is a full and adequate account of the typical course of these histories, their chief constituents and stages, and the factors shaping and determining their course
(iv) in the pursuit of these aims, the approach of psychology must not only be *dynamic* and *causal*, like that of all other natural sciences, but also, because of the special character of its subject-matter, *contextual* and *functional*, *historical* and *genetic*.[1]

In other words, all specific psychological facts and happenings occur in particular contexts and at particular periods in cumulative individual psychic life-histories. They cannot be properly described and understood except as elements of these. Psychology has to lay bare the structure, interdependences and successive unfolding of these histories as integral wholes ; and the facts of our cognitive life and activities, all the history of our learning and knowing, can only be grasped as living parts of this total pattern. They share its characters, are in continual interrelation and interaction with the rest, make their own vital contribution to the course of each history, but are in turn sustained, shaped and given their significance by the rest.

(3) The above statement may seem to raise, or to raise again, one large question, which calls for a further word of preliminary comment.

The normal way of describing individual human life-histories in objective language would obviously be as histories of cumulative

---

[1] The full meanings of these terms will be developed in the later exposition. The sense in which the approach of all the other natural sciences is dynamic and causal (whether or not these terms are used) is, I think, implicit in their methods, manifest throughout their history and demonstrated by the very existence of all their technological and practical applications. See also Chapter VI on the notion of Causality.

interaction with a given physical environment or outside world. Their main refrain is a constant alternation of undergoing and doing, doing and undergoing. Learning and knowing appear as primarily a particular type of effect of undergoing, which occurs under certain conditions ; an effect that endures and becomes cumulative and can only be depicted as the *progressive registration of undergoing-patterns*, leading to the building up of prepared, advance " doing " patterns in readiness for any recurrent similar undergoings. We shall be more fully concerned with this process shortly. The present point is that our psychology does seem not merely to require but wholly to rest upon the postulate of a physical world around the organic human individual, with which he is in this relation of cumulative interaction that shapes his history.

But the answer is that just psychology, of all sciences, is most clearly not dependent on that postulate. Whatever else we may believe our " physical world " to be, there is certainly no specifiable feature of it or aspect of it which has not *also* the status of a psychological content, or element in our psychic history. Whether we have come to know or think about it through direct perception or through human report or even through inference down to the most abstruse kind, the mere fact that we know or think about it testifies to its place within our history, and by the same token raises the empirical-psychological questions when and how it entered into our history. For everything we believe or know, we must have learnt, or come to believe or know, at some time in our experience-history. (Even if we assume, by way of limiting case, the existence of innate ideas or innate knowledge, there will be some date or phase when we first discovered that we had these ideas or knowledge, i.e. when they entered our conscious *experience*-history as such, in this explicit, realised shape.)

Thus there can be no inherent difficulty in telling our psychological story in purely psychological or experiential terms ; in fact we cannot use any terms which, whatever we may commonly suppose to the contrary, do not start off with such a meaning first of all. This is not indeed the whole story ; the course of our experience leads us progressively to assign a special status to certain kinds of experience-contents, and when we use our objective language we are affirming that status and a vast deal which gets built upon it and around it. But, as we have just affirmed, this is itself an outcome of our experience-history, and we can therefore the more confidently undertake to put the latter in terms which begin by assuming nothing else. In effect, the entire cycle of alternation of undergoing and doing, doing and under-going which we should commonly describe as the history of our cumulative interaction with the outside world can just as readily, and with a more fundamental accuracy, be stated as a history of alternation and cumulative interaction of different kinds of experiences with one another.

For the rest, our description must now be left to tell its own tale.

CHAPTER III

EXPERIENTIAL BASIS FOR THE DISTINCTION BE-TWEEN TRUTH AND FALSITY. THE DYNAMICS OF EXPANDING KNOWLEDGE AND GROWING LOGIC

I.—SOME BASIC WORKING DISTINCTIONS WITHIN OUR EXPERIENCE

(1) In this section we are only concerned to sketch in very lightly certain early experienced distinctions within our total experience which our later history shows to be fundamental. They will be further developed in their appropriate places, but it seems desirable to present them in broad outline in advance.

There are various pervasive qualitative distinctions which cannot but impress themselves cumulatively on the child from his first few weeks onwards. In the light of the way in which they sort themselves out later on, we can set down something like the following main groups of experiences (which of course happen in constant interaction with one another, as elements in a single progressive story) :

    (i) Affective-conative

    (ii) Receptive-perceptual

    (iii) Active, differentiated later into :

        (a) attentional
        (b) locomotive
        (c) operative

    (iv) Cognitive, rapidly differentiated into :

        (a) recognitive
        (b) anticipative
        (c) representative.

The whole way in which each of these basic kinds of experience presents itself, i.e. not only its own quality but all its setting and affiliations, demarcates it more and more clearly and sharply from each of the other kinds (whilst at the same time bringing its own different sub-species more and more closely together into one cognate group). " Affective-conative " experiences are first of all those experiences which carry a strong charge of excitement and nisus towards or away ; presently they also become peculiarly bound up with the child's developing sense of himself as a subject (the focal " I " that feels and strives), and with the perceptual and active experience-focus he calls his own body. " Receptive-perceptual " experiences come to the child as a more or less neutral filling in and background for those other, far more agitating happenings ; moreover they occur with the very distinctive character of fields with foci in them, they link up in special ways with attentional experiences on the one hand and cognitive ones on the other, and they grow together cumulatively in larger and larger contexts. " Active " experiences have a *sui generis* quality of energy, and at the same time of sustained and directed tension, which stands in sharp contrast to the " undergoing " or passive tenor characteristic of most of the others, indeed initially of all of them. The class of experiences we have called cognitive distinguish themselves from the rest not only by their direct experienced quality, but by a peculiar feature which is crucial for our approach and to which we must now turn more specifically.

(2) This feature is essentially that they come to us as derivative and secondary. By comparison with them, all other experiences can be called primary. (We also often speak of *immediate* or *direct* experiencing, especially in relation to perception, in the sense of direct apprehension of and contact with a reality other than ourselves ; but this is best avoided, not only because it begs the question we are here setting out to answer,[1] but also because in an equally good sense recognising or remembering are just as truly distinctive modes of immediate experiencing as perceiving or feeling.)

Whether we happen to be right or wrong in any particular application, the *character* of an experience of recognition is : " this-before," or " something-like-this-before." Similarly, the character of an experience of expectation is " something-like-before-now-coming." The similar element in a remembrance or recollection or representation is self-evident ; imagining or fantasying are special derivatives from the same stem, which turn away from direct or avowed derivativeness but still carry enough of this about them as a rule to leave no doubt about their origin.

The distinction between primary and derivative experience-modes will be found pivotal not only for our account of truth and falsity but for our psychology of knowledge in general. It will be noted that receptive-perceptual experiences are *not* placed in the cognitive class. This would in fact again be question-begging, and quite gratuitously so. Whilst for the purposes of description we have had to use our later psychologists' labels, the suggestion here is in essence that, from a very early stage, in virtue of their direct experienced qualitative differences and affiliations, the foregoing main groupings *establish and segregate themselves*, of their own momentum, as separate functional systems. But it is not in the least necessary, from our point of view, to claim that the experiences we later call perceptual carry within them intrinsically any peculiar character which directly marks them out as cognitive in their own right. We can in fact easily demonstrate the way in which this character *accrues to them in the course of experience*, precisely through their experienced relation to everything else in our history, but above all to those other types of occurrence we have distinguished as cognitive (in virtue of their special quality of derivativeness from and reference forward to other experiences).

(3) Finally, for the purposes of our later exposition, we must take the theme of our " cognitive " class of experiences one important stage further. Recognition implies retention and revival. The occurrence of anticipation or expectation shows that this process goes far beyond single experience-contents or qualities. A fundamental fact of our history is that there is such a thing as the psychic *cohesion* of the diverse parts or elements of our experience, so that revival tends to be not merely of something similar to a given primary experience-content, but also of other contents which have previously occurred (usually a number of times) in close conjunction or combination with the directly revived one and have become linked and co-retained with it.

This may seem suspiciously reminiscent of the well-worn formula of associationism, but before it is assumed to be open to the familiar objections to the latter, our earlier emphasis on the perceptual *field* should be remembered. The key-concept is in fact that of tried, tested and consolidated linkage, in coherent contexts, in the place of mere habitual atomic association. What degrees and kinds of such linkage are possible and what can be made of them, within the framework of a cumulative experience-history which expressly insists on our full life of feeling, learning and action, should not be prejudged, but should be left to be shown.

II.—THE PRIMARY EXPERIENTIAL BASIS FOR THE DISTINCTION BETWEEN TRUTH AND FALSITY

(4) Our first task is to focus full attention on a very commonplace situation or occurrence, to which we have already alluded.

In some of its aspects it has indeed long figured prominently in philosophical discussion, but nevertheless its rightful significance has largely been missed. It has not been seen *through*, in all its implications and consequences ; it has not been viewed as it needs to be, functionally, contextually and historically, nor appreciated as the great parting of the ways which in fact it is. It is a situation which begins to happen within the first week or two of our experience and then goes on happening continually, but with a capacity for the most radical divergences of outcome which in turn have the most far-reaching, inevitable and cumulative results.

This situation or experience is that of recognition, with anticipation or expectation. We all know well how easily and simply it can be brought about ; indeed, behaviouristic evidence of it (in the shape of unmistakable pre-adjustments) has been found in infants down to ten days old. In more or less associationist language, (i) repetitions of similar primary experience-constellations (or sometimes even a single very vivid one) lead to (ii) the *recognition* of any further experience similar to part (a sufficient part) of that constellation, together with (iii) the *revival* or re-experiencing of the rest, and (iv) the (automatic, mostly behaviouristic and implicit) *expectation* of its actual *recurrence* (i.e. as another similar *primary* experience-constellation).

The foregoing has been stated in somewhat careful terms, which avoid certain time-honoured traps ; but even so the description may not be sufficiently guarded yet. We cannot in effect be too careful about what it is which is recognised, what it is that is revived, and what it is that is expected. Normally we talk, and think, of recognising objects (or happenings or states of affairs, etc.) ; recalling this or that fact usually associated with them ; and so being led to expect to find the same fact again. But that of course takes a vast deal for granted and belongs to a comparatively advanced level of belief and judgment. When we are seeking not to take anything for granted (beyond the occurrence of our experiences as experiences), we are still left with all the characteristic features and the characteristic alternative courses of our recognition-revival-expectation situations, but now in terms only of actual psychic contents and of the vital *experienced* distinction between primary and derivative experiencing.

What in effect happens is that particular primary experiences (above all of the kind we later label perceptual) evoke in us, as it seems almost concurrently, the further distinctive experience of *recognition*, plus the equally characteristic experience of *expectation or anticipation*. This latter remains for the most part behaviouristic and implicit ; but in so far as it becomes more explicit and articulate, it divides in turn into two distinct aspects, first of all of a not-primary *derivative* experience, or re-experiencing or revival, and, secondly, of a unique *tension towards* the field of the initial primary " recognised " experience, a preparing for the derivative one to be taken up and absorbed into a coming *like but primary* experience.

We can watch this sort of sequence in ourselves a hundred times a day ; we can follow it back in our memory as far back as this will reach ; we can see *all* the typical signs and accompaniments and outcomes of it in infants certainly down to their first few months : the smile or grimace of recognition, the preparation and tension, and the obvious experience of consummation . . . or of complete surprise and discomfiture. And we have only to appreciate, with the help of every sort of supporting evidence, that such series of occurrences (depending on nothing but repetitions of mutually similar experience-constellations) do recur continually from almost the beginning of our individual life-histories, to find that we are furnished with a most powerful and pregnant key to most of the mysteries of truth and error, of reality and mere belief, and indeed to our whole cognitive development.

(5) The point is surely this : the expectations which are evoked in and through recognition are expectations of further experiences (of the same *primary* type) to come. Past ones are revived or incipiently re-experienced, in a secondary, derivative way ; but because of their very evocation by the *given* primary experience, they remain attached to this and are projected forward, in a unique way, into the next moment of time, with the expectancy that the same experiences will now happen in their fresh, primary form again. And then in fact more primary experience does come ; and mostly it takes up the waiting re-experience or pre-experience and, as it were, re-mints it in its fresh, primary mode. But quite often the primary experiencing which actually comes does not do this ; it first sharply collides with the waiting pre-experience, and then overwhelms it—breaks it up and puts itself in its place.

This again is something which we can watch in ourselves almost any day ; mostly on a small scale, but all too frequently also on a large one. We can follow it back as far as our memory will reach, and we can observe all the gamut of its expressions in infants in their first year. Surprise, disappointment, discomfiture, confusion, fear : the combination speaks for itself with irresistible eloquence. We can in fact also see how inevitable this sort of débâcle is, precisely in the earlier stages of automatic expectation-formation. The young child establishes his linkages of certain sets of experiences either by just a few repetitions or even by one or two vivid and impressive occurrences ; but everything we later learn goes to show that linkages thus formed are only too apt to lead to error, i.e. to false expectation, and so to the dramatic experience of expectation actually falsified.

(6) Our suggestion now is that it is the *relation* between expectations of primary experiences to come (usually evoked by given such experiences but always going beyond them) and those that do actually come, which is the first and controlling psychological basis for our distinction between truth and falsity. That is to say, it is this relation, itself continually experienced in either its positive or its negative form, which gives their fundamental *correlative* meanings to both these notions.

The negative form is far and away the more distinctive and illuminating one ; the positive is mostly just not noticed at all because, so long as the pattern of further primary experiences fits into the developing expectation-pattern and absorbs this, we pass straight on in our course towards our aims or purposes of the moment. But obviously we can at any time also pay attention to the positive type of experience and take cognisance of its every detail ; we do so pre-eminently in scientific experiments, where we expressly formulate our expectations beforehand in the most precise terms, and then watch minutely to see whether or not they are fulfilled.

Our own attention here will be chiefly focused on the negative class, for reasons which will explain themselves. But we begin with the common crux of both.

(7) What we have here, in effect, is the most evident and unquestionable relation of *correspondence* or *non-correspondence*. Everyone is familiar with the difficulties which the so-called " naïve " correspondence theory of truth gets into, and the many different directions in which philosophers have struck out in search of a more tenable position, from endeavours to save the name of the theory at the expense of most of its " naïve " substance (e.g., through the notion of correspondence of structure or order), up to the extreme " coherence " view. The most obvious difficulty lies of course in jumping the apparent transcendent or metaphysical gap between our would-be " knowledge " and the

" reality " it claims to know : what *other* way have we of getting at the latter, beyond that very would-be knowledge, the veridicity or " correspondence " of which is at issue ?

This is not the place for a detailed critical consideration of the traditional philosophic approach to the problem, or supposed problem ; we need only comment very briefly, firstly, that this approach has been vitiated at the outset by the absence of a preliminary empirical psycho-linguistic study of the *terms used*, and secondly that the endless vicious circle of argument shifting to and fro between questions of word-meaning and questions of fact might have been broken at any time by closer attention to our actual experiences of *non*-correspondence which so impressively tell their own tale.

Our present object is to bring into full relief what they have to say. And in the first place, there is no metaphysical difficulty here about the notion of correspondence. We remain wholly within the realm of experience. We start off with the mode of revival-with-expectation, and we go on (in the most important class of cases) to the primary mode we call perception. And we find that the perceptual experience which actually comes to us often carries with it a direct, acute, specific experience of clash, or non-correspondence, with our previous expectation-state, with the most vivid and dramatic accompaniments and further consequences. This is an experience which we can examine and study, in a myriad of varied examples which illuminate in turn every aspect and every implication of it.

In the second place now, we may note that although there is here no philosophic or metaphysical transcendence, there *is* transcendence of a very real kind. The correspondence we are dealing with (whether it so dramatically fails to happen, or whether it just smoothly happens) is not of the static or quasi-spatial type usually envisaged, but is *temporal*. It is, however, precisely this character which generates its own most pregnant form of transcendence. Our expectation is of a further primary (usually perceptual) experience to come (an evoked re-experience projected forward in time as a pre-experience) ; but in virtue of this very fact it is directed to a moment in time which, at the moment of the expectation, has not happened yet, a moment which is outside our experience, our life, our history so far ; which —as we often and all too convincingly find—stands in a relation of transcending reality to us. But then this further moment of time *happens* and a further primary experience *comes to us* ; only, it proves to be something quite different from what we had projected ahead of us, it thrusts right through what we had expected or " thought " or " believed," overpowers this and seizes its place. Our anti-expected new experience crashes in, and just by doing so becomes an independent, superior, controlling reality. Moreover, by that very process, and, as it were, in the same breath, it both *overturns* and *defines* what was there before, as something wrongly believed, something merely inward or merely expected or thought or believed, and so believed *in error*. What does all this, however, is still just another *experience* ; but now one with a new overriding status and significance, an experience representative of what really is there, i.e. of *what is the fact*, as distinct from and opposed to what we merely imagined.

III.—DYNAMICS OF EXPANDING KNOWLEDGE AND GROWING LOGIC

(8) It will be clear that this is only a very condensed and telescoped description of something that does not emerge from or depend upon a single experience, or even a series of repetitions of one and the same kind of experience, but upon a continual cumulative process of recurrence of similar experiences in the most diverse forms and settings, all confirming, consolidating and extending one another. We can find all the characteristic features in every individual case, and we can readily see that the essential relation between expectation and actual experience is exactly the same even in all our cases of successful correspondence (if we stop to attend to them). But the burden and significance of the relation is only borne in upon us progressively as we go on experiencing it in all its different forms, and though it plays the most fundamental part in our whole *working* organisation of our experience and world, we may never reach the stage of getting that part fully articulated. There is in fact far more consciousness of the meaning of the relation, above all in its immensely revealing negative form, embodied in literature, the drama, biography and history than in our traditional philosophic thinking. Again, few of us are unaware in practice of the extent to which a single unexpected new experience may destroy an entire previous system of beliefs and assumptions and a way of life based on these—and may compel us to build our world anew (if we remain there to do so). Whilst any close attention to our history as a history brings out the great pervasive pattern of learning and growth by which, as we live forward in time, we are constantly forming and projecting ahead of us and around us, from earliest childhood, both

endless specific expectations and larger (mainly implicit) expectation-schemes on every sort of scale, up to our generalised world-
picture ; and we are continually building our schemes of purposes, plans, desires, hopes and action on them. But at the same
time we are incessantly compelled to correct, modify and reconstruct most of these structures, on every sort of scale, from the
most local to the most general, in the light of new and better
learning ; in other words, in the light of new primary experiences
which impose themselves on us and enforce the readjustment of
our previous thought-structures to them. We accept all this as a
matter of course ; the primacy of our primary experience is the
first great lesson we learn from our experience ; it signifies the
" reality outside ourselves," and more powerful than ourselves,
which we have to take in and to which we have to adapt. The
main movement of all our learning-history from infancy to adulthood consists in fact of the alternating formation, correction and
transcendence of progressively wider expectation-schemes and
expectation-horizons ; and our later adult learning-history, in
so far as we continue to have one, individually or collectively, is
no different. We take, indeed, the greatest care to absorb and
apply the moral in our empirical science, which, for that reason
more than for any other, *is* progressive and cumulative science.

Our suggestion here is that this immensely powerful and
ubiquitous *vera causa* forms a major experiential source and
foundation of the special status we assign to our perceptual
experience, and indeed of the whole distinction between inner
and outer, between " merely " subjective and objective actuality.
But it must be emphasised that it is far from being the only
source ; our main psychological thesis is that the tremendous
felt force and reality of the distinction rests precisely upon the
convergence of a large number of independent but mutually
supporting and reinforcing orders of experience. The peculiar
relation of *dependence* of our expectations (anticipations of primary
experience) on the actual primary experiences which come to
us, and above all the way in which this dependence is dramatically
brought home to us in every case of falsification of expectation, is
only one of the above orders of experience, even if it is a specially
pregnant one. Some of the other chief orders will form the
themes of our later sections. The important point, if we wish
really to understand the psychological basis, the strength and the
intrinsic unshakeableness, of our " naïve " belief in our common
sense world, is to form an adequate view of the entire inter-

supporting structure of different experience-orders on which it rests and which in effect it affirms and " means."

(9) We cannot attempt here to work out the full bearings of our expectation-history, which in effect would involve the whole history of our experience, our beliefs, our knowledge and indeed of our psychic life. All we can do is to call closer attention to those features of the key-situation of falsified expectation which in turn bring out most clearly the part it is destined to play, virtually day by day, in our total cognitive development.

(i) The processes by which, from our first few weeks, both specific and general expectations are formed and extended are mostly such that, as we have seen, they positively court a high proportion of errors. We have already referred to the effect of mere repetition or even mere vividness in forming associative bonds ; we might now add that, in so far as these bonds begin by operating successfully, (*a*) they go on spreading by analogy, i.e. they are apt to be touched off by less and less appropriate stimuli (*b*) they are set off by smaller and smaller segments of stimulus (*c*) they go on extending their own span. All these are trends which mean riding for a fall, and sooner or later getting it.

(ii) The failure or falsification of a fully-held expectation or expectation-scheme is most often, at the best, a somewhat disagreeable experience, which carries with it *some* degree of jar and discomfiture, and often a severe degree. (The most notable exception, which proves the rule, is the way in which we learn to *play* at it, and so to assert our mastery of it, in carefully circumscribed settings and above all in the verbal form of jokes.) We are stopped in our course, confused and, at least momentarily, made helpless.

(iii) Very often the same failure or falsification brings in its train actual hurt, danger, disappointment and frustration. These may be of any degree, up to catastrophe. All our prepared apparatus of adaptation and appropriate action breaks down, and anything may happen before we can rally, or we may just get no chance of doing so.

(iv) On every sort of ground, therefore, these experiences act as a strong stimulus. Even where in their immediate impact they are comparatively slight and unimportant, they carry with them at least an undertone of " something wrong " and some reminder of what this *might* lead to. In any event even their least impact tends to evoke an immediate, virtually automatic attempt at readjustment. Some rule or assumption which has hitherto worked out successfully has suddenly failed : where are we now ? What do we do next ?—In important cases (though not in the extreme ones, in which we are too overwhelmed) we are thrown into a direct struggle to cope with the situation, to sort ourselves out, to get rid of the wrong expectation-scheme and see if we can quickly substitute the (or an) appropriate one. Or if it is too late for this, we struggle at least to find out what has gone wrong, so that we can avoid the same pitfall or mistake the next time.

(v) The great variety of our experiences of falsified expectation provides us with every degree and every combination both of active motive and of learning opportunity. The experience as such tends to light up both the previous situation and its own impact on this. The expectation, from being automatic and just taken for granted, is turned into something conscious and realised. And this process brings into focus the various elements of the structure of expectation-situations, with the high light sometimes on this, sometimes on that constituent. Thus we are taught to become progressively aware of that structure, both in particular cases and as a general guiding fact.

(vi) The basic structural features so brought into the limelight are obviously, at the outset, these two : first, the immediate stimulus, the actual piece of primary experiencing, which has started our particular expectation off ; then, the latter itself, the re-experiencing which, when so started off, projects itself as a pre-experiencing of the next primary experience to come. If this, when it actually comes, collides with our expectation and shatters it, our startled attention is first of all forced back (where the situation permits) to the primary experience-content from which it all began. Very often it will in fact still be available or recoverable. Quite often there will now be more of it (a larger field). And it may well happen that even if it is still recognisably a similar, or partly similar, experience to that which originally started us off, it is now sufficiently different to evoke quite another set of expectations, which are therefore, by the next further primary experience, fulfilled.

We are indeed increasingly confronted with two alternative and widely divergent courses of readjustment. It is easiest to state these clearly in our later object-language, the more so since they do not assume explicit shape till a certain amount of progress has been made, along our other lines of advance, towards the organisation of our experience in terms of objects and an objective world. But again these alternative courses, in the very process by which they make themselves felt, contribute towards that organisation, and help to articulate and confirm our picture of the objective order of things.

What happens is in effect that the child finds himself forming two main differing types of expectation-patterns within the field of his perceptual experience. We shall be more fully concerned with this process in our next section, but since our psychic life is a single cumulative history, we cannot move very far in any one direction without having also to draw on what has meanwhile been going on in others. Anticipating, therefore, to some extent, we must say that the child's experience has been sorting itself out into, on the one hand, a wide range of *co-recurring* and highly cohesive perceptual constellations, and on the other a variety of *successive* perceptual patterns grouped round these co-recurring nuclei or foci, controlled by them and evoked through them. In other words, given perceptual experiences very often start up, *in the first place*, the larger expectation-pattern corresponding to one of these kinds of foci, and it is this pattern which then (often in conjunction with further perceptual experiences) sets off in turn another expectation-sequence already linked with it in our thought.

In consequence of this developing organisation, we may easily find, and frequently do, that the very first recoil from a falsified *specific* expectation towards the activating primary experience shows that it was the controlling initial expectation-pattern which was already wrong. In other words, we had made an error of recognition ; we had assumed or inferred (from the first perceptual stimulus) the wrong *kind* of object. Our further specific expectation has therefore not been shown false in itself, i.e. in its relation to the kind of object to which it properly belongs ; it has rather been shown to have been misapplied and to be irrelevant. Of course our error of " recognition " is still, strictly and properly speaking, one of expectation ; in our ordinary summary language, we speak of recognising objects, but what we really mean by this is recognising some particular piece of primary (perceptual) experiencing as an *indication of the presence* of a particular type of object. And that, again, in full experience-language means recognising that piece of primary experiencing as familiar and having it evoke in us the *expectation*-pattern of a constellation of further primary experiences which together make up our picture, or a substantial part of our picture, of that type of object. An error of recognition signifies simply that the wrong constellation of expectations has been activated, and that it will be duly (as a rule very quickly) falsified.

This is all in line with the processes we have already described and introduces no new difficulties or complications (except in so far as we fail to provide the proper historical background for our language). The significant point here is merely the very distinctive bifurcation of our experiences of falsified expectations into what we find to be errors of recognition (usually fairly readily corrected and for the most part with only limited repercussions), and what we find to be genuine errors of generalised belief. For in the measure in which the former crystallise out as such, we are left the more clearly and sharply with all those cases where our return to the evoking stimulus provides no such way out, but *confirms* our recognitive expectations and confronts us with the fact that it is our linkage of that class of objects with that particular belief or expectation about them which is undependable and wrong.

(vii) The first effect then is to inhibit the automaticity of this expectation or belief ; to teach us that instead of our assumed " always " we must work on an at least provisional " sometimes, but sometimes not," or " some, but not all." But if anything of importance to us is involved, we obviously cannot stop there but must try, if at all possible, to find some way of distinguishing " when " from " when not." The easiest way naturally, where the circumstances favour, is to break up our one previous recognitive-expectation-pattern into *two*, clearly distinct from one another, so that we can keep our original further expectation or belief attached with full confidence to one of these, and detach it completely from the other. But too often we fail in this, and whilst sometimes we can establish other means of separating or somehow demarcating the two kinds of case, we have also to content ourselves with being left with a vast number of " some-but-not-all and we can't be sure which " beliefs. These then demand their own mixture of alertness and inhibition, which anyhow is vastly better than either complete ignorance or blind and mainly wrong belief.

(viii) The foregoing is no more than the most schematic summary of a vast number of occurrences and processes taking place over a wide front in cumulative interaction over a long period. When we consider that both the processes of expectation-formation and those of evocation of particular expectations and interaction between them and our actual primary experiences are going on practically every moment of the waking life of every child from his first few weeks throughout the rest of his history, it should be clear that there is the amplest scope for most of the permutations and combinations of the dynamics of that inter-action to work themselves out. It is not difficult, in effect, to see how much of the basic structure of our later adult knowledge and adult logic is already implicit—and indeed quite soon largely explicit—in the elementary experiences and processes we have described.

Thus even the most rudimentary expectation-situation contains in principle all the essential features of the applicative syllogism. The evocative primary experience or stimulus fulfils the function of the minor premise ; the activated linkage, or associative bond, or "repeating universal" constitutes the functional major premise ; the specific expectation here and now (in virtue of that bond) of a particular kind of primary experience to come, is the conclusion. And as this is instantly tested and, where wrong, all too forcibly rebutted, and we are applying the same functional-inferential procedure all day long, we are very tellingly started on our road to a less automatic and more searching attitude both towards the separate factors and to the logic of their *relation* within the basic inferential pattern.

This road leads eventually to immense complexities, insidious aberrations and outcomes which, when considered in abstract isolation, appear to be quite unrelated to the starting-points we have described. The contention here is that, if only we realised the cumulative historical character of the entire process, and thus of even its most remote and refined end-products, and if we followed the evolution of these through stage by stage, they would fall into their rightful place and we should be saved from the endless false mysteries (and pseudo-solutions) which arise from our traditional a-historical approach to historical pro-ducts.

(ix) The process cannot be worked out more fully within the present limits of space, but we may end this chapter by noting several points about its most developed phase which provide striking confirmation of the crucial and enduring significance of the elementary situations we have picked out.

(a) The recognitive-predicative structure is broadly retained throughout the growth of our empirical scientific knowledge. This is organised in the main in terms of particular classes of objects (of attention and inquiry), *which are unequivocally recognisable or identifiable in their appropriate fields of occurrence* ; and it consists of bodies of systematic information *about* these classes. To quite a large extent indeed the latter are classes of objects in the simplest and most " naïve " sense of the word (animals, plants, rocks, celestial bodies, bodies and particles at rest and in motion). But of course the principle is not altered if for " naïve " objects we substitute, as we have done, objects (or subjects) of attention and inquiry, so long as their presence is unequivocally recognisable or identifiable. That is, so long as we can specify or describe a constellation of primary experiences (i.e., formulate a representation-pattern or expectation-pattern) such that, at any time when we actually experience or could actually experience that constellation, we should regard ourselves as in the presence of " objects " of that class. Thus the subject-matter of a science may be a class of substances, or a type of event or process or even relation, but we shall still have a controlling nucleus of recognitive specification, and then a corpus of information *about* the class of event or whatever it may be, identified by means of the recognitive nucleus. (This corpus may include fundamental information about the ultimate character, make-up, or as we say nature, of the subject-matter itself ; but we shall still need an ordinary, plain recognitive specification for the absolutely vital purpose of telling us when *we are*, and when *we are not*, in its presence.)

(*b*) The above structure is in effect necessitated by the principle of fact-control on which all our empirical scientific knowledge is based. It is the one assured way of avoiding the fatal see-saw between debates about word-meanings and debates about substantive beliefs in which philosophic thought has become caught. A clear and unequivocal reference to a determinate " objective " field or class of entities, under the control of which we can place ourselves and which can thus become a source of recognitive, of exploratory and of verificatory (or falsifying) *primary* experience is the only means of building up bodies of cumulative tested information or science. The reference points the sole way both for the gathering of data and for the testing of generalisations and inferences, hypotheses and theories. But that it may do so effectively, it is clearly essential that we should be able to distinguish between the question of the *presence* of the *subject-matter*, and the *truth or otherwise* of anything that may be affirmed or suggested *about it*. Scientific fact-control of inferences and theories and beliefs generally consists in identifying the presence of the subject-matter, in suitably selected test instances, and then examining whether what is affirmed or suggested holds good or not.[1] Hence the essential nature of the distinction between recognitive and predicative knowledge. (This is quite compatible with the fact that as our predicative knowledge grows, we tend to shift the line between it and our " recognitive " information and to transfer no little of the former to the latter division, so that our *strictly* recognitive information becomes merely ancillary. What is essential is simply that the dividing line *at any one time* should be clear and agreed, that only fully established knowledge should be transferred, and that the recognitive information actually used to identify the presence of the appropriate subject-matter at a given time should be entirely unequivocal.)

(*c*) In our scientific procedure more than anywhere else we have learnt the full lesson of our proneness to premature and excessive generalisation ; we assume that almost any unconditional general proposition is almost certainly wrong, and we go to every sort of trouble we can think of to uncover its latent errors, conditions or limitations. And our final test is of course direct observation (preferably after experiment), applied to the actual controlling subject-matter, in the most widely varied or most unpromising circumstances possible. In other words, we try to get our beliefs more nearly right by doing everything possible to prove them wrong (unlike philosophy, in which we apply every resource of logical ingenuity to *protect* them from being shown wrong).

(*d*) Finally, when we want to carry out our most searching tests on any generalisation or inference, hypothesis or theory, our procedure is precisely that by which we are first taught the nature and the meaning of fact-control and by which all our first involuntary errors are brought home to us. We formulate a specific expectation (prediction or deduction from the theorem under test) applicable in a specific set of circumstances ; we carry out the appropriate set of observations or experiments in that set of circumstances ; and we compare what we find with our theoretical expectation. In other words, we test the latter deliberately, by the appropriate primary experience, for correspondence or non-correspondence, in just the way which our own

---

[1] The above may not appear to cover *existential* beliefs or theories, but these of course are simply cases of specifying sufficiently clearly what it is that is asserted to exist and in what objective, i.e., *controlling*, field of existence. Science has no difficulty over these requirements, and can apply the same fact-control to existential propositions as to predicative propositions about any class of existents. Philosophic difficulties arise chiefly through vagueness, ambiguity and shiftingness, which evade or preclude *any* sort of control.

personal history has always willy-nilly forced on us. And, generally speaking, we regard *non*-correspondence as negatively decisive, whilst correspondence is as a rule, even under the most exacting conditions, viewed only as strongly supporting. The support is of course strongest in the case of a crucial experiment where we believe we can refine our choice down to two alternative theories which would give different pre-definable results in a given case, and we can then examine and compare the case. But the vital point is always the comparison between something actually found (experienced in the primary mode) and something previously specified as what one *would find* (anticipative representation of such experience) if a certain general proposition (linkage of experience-contents or findings) held good or were true. That is our initial psychic truth-falsity situation, and that remains our most final and definitive scientific truth-falsity test.

(*e*) By way of supplementary note, we may remark that the foregoing is the simplest answer to all those who decry the notion of correspondence on psychological grounds, such as the supposed facts of imageless thought, the difficulties of formulating general images or representations, etc. The plain truth is that the comparison of thoughts with facts must be capable of being made, because it *is* constantly being made—on all levels of thought up to the most advanced scientific. The supposed psychological difficulties are in effect mostly philosophic red herrings. We largely forestall them if we are careful to appreciate in advance that the comparison of " thoughts " with " facts " is actually always a comparison of re-experiencings, or of products, even if at some remove, of such re-experiencings, with primary experience *of the same kind*. (We are comparing like with like.) We cannot pursue the subject in psychological detail here, but the test is what happens precisely in our crucial scientific experiments. And quite generally, scientific fact-control is only possible, and natural science only exists, because we can always formulate in advance what, on any given *scientific* view, we should expect to find (in the form of primary experience), in such a way that we can directly *compare* this with what we do find (in the form of the same kind of primary experience) ; and because moreover we can usually pronounce, not only on broad correspondence or non-correspondence, but on their precise degree.[1]

---

[1] It will be noted that the above standpoint comes very close again in many respects to the position expressed by the Logical Positivists in their Principle of Verifiability. I should agree in fact that the latter affirms a vital truth, though it has often been formulated and defended in unfortunate and imperfectly justifiable ways. But, once

(10) Before leaving this sketch it seems desirable to bring out, if only to acknowledge its incompleteness, a few of the more significant ways in which it has over-simplified the experiential picture :

(i) In our sharp antithesis between non-correspondence and correspondence we have chiefly focused on the more extreme cases of the former. But whilst there are abundant instances of these, it is important for the full psychological story to recognise also all the partial correspondences, or partial non-correspondences, and all the variations in *degree* of non-correspondence or correspondence (from barely noticed divergence right down to the most startling disparity) which we continually meet. These do not alter the main structure we have outlined ; but they introduce into it a variety of secondary but significant modulations which cannot here be pursued. To take only one example : our constant experience of minor degrees of non-correspondence with expectation-patterns formed from some few previous cases leads us to broaden these patterns by a range, or at any rate a fringe, of *normal variations*. Some of the traits characteristic of a class of things (events, processes, etc.) fluctuate ; some are not characteristic, just because they so commonly and widely fluctuate. Our expectation-patterns have constantly to be accommodated to the sort of world we find, not only by sharp correction and reconstruction, but also by a general acquisition of varying degrees of *habitual* flexibility in different sorts of context. Yet it remains true that they fail of their whole purpose and value unless they retain a core of determinateness on which we can definitely rely and build—build further knowledge and build growing schemes of action in so far as they prove dependably true (which always, however, means also : are capable of being shown false).

(ii) From incomplete or imperfect correspondences of the above type we must clearly distinguish certain *mixtures* of correspondence and non-correspondence which present some of the acutest challenges to our existing expectation-beliefs. Rules which have become strongly established by apparent regular compliance seem suddenly flouted : everything indicates a case where they *should* apply, and yet they fail. This is a theme which we need barely touch upon here, because we shall return to it in Chapter

---

more, what seems to me essential is to provide the full psychological background and context, in a way which the Logical Positivists do not merely neglect, but reject as not relevant. If they were *Psychological* Positivists. . . .

VII, which indeed very generally takes up again the tale of the present section.

(iii) To avoid needless complications we have not considered in any very specific way a great class of experiences which have functionally much in common with those of sharp non-correspondence and indeed merge into these, but which have also a very distinctive character and range of their own. This class is that of unexpected findings, as distinct from anti-expected ones. " Unexpected " means unprepared for, and can be as disconcerting and disturbing and hurtful and dangerous as anything that directly clashes with a specific expectation. On the other hand, at the other end of the range there are many kinds of situation in which we *expect* (generically) the unexpected, or at any rate are not taken by surprise by it : e.g., if we enter into a new environment or start exploring an unfamiliar range of experiences, etc., etc. Here again, however, it will usually be true that we only expect a certain *degree* of unexpectedness, or at any rate gradually learn to expect this ; that is, no magic or miracles or fairy tale happenings, but only unusually wide variations within our set familiar patterns. The key lies of course in our progressive formation of broad generic expectation-schemes : schemes of what *may* happen in a given kind of situation or context, as well as what will ; schemes of the general character and scope of whole local contexts (the child's—or adult's—home setting, street, town, part of the country ; familiar human relationships, plant world, animal world, mechanical world, and so on). The main correctness and sufficiency of these generic patterns can be as important to the child as the truth of specific determinate expectations ; anything he encounters which he is quite unprepared for may, as we have said, offer him as much of a menace, as well as surprise, as any anti-expected experience.

That again is a topic which will recur to some extent when in Chapter VII we take up the wider theme of Explanation.

(11) It should be noted, in conclusion, that whilst the present sketch is far removed from utilising all the material which is already available to us (if only we will pay attention to it), there is also room and need for a vast deal more of specific *new* empirical inquiry and research. We require this indeed before we can fill in the *precise* steps and stages of some of our most important cognitive advances. The proper empirical psychology of knowledge, claiming its whole ground and carrying out the right field-inquiries in regard to all its key topics, is still at an early stage

of its growth. It is true that with so much that is fully accessible and clear, we need have no difficulty about a rough general sketch-map showing the main lay-out and dominant features of our field ; but the detailed ordnance survey is still mostly to come.

IV.—SUPPLEMENTARY NOTE ABOUT THE TERMS " KNOWING," " KNOWLEDGE," AND " COGNITION "

(12) Whilst by and large our chief word-meanings are to be filled in by the actual content and structure of the psychological picture we are building up, the welter of confusions round the crucial terms " knowing " and " knowledge " seems to call for at least a preliminary key. This will draw to a considerable extent on what has already been set out, but also depends largely on what is still to follow, and can therefore only be regarded as a provisional guide.

We must, then, distinguish the following chief elements of meaning of the term " knowing," each of them often used separately, in certain ranges of context, but most or all of them frequently compounded together in one shifting and elusive muddle :

(1) To be aquainted or familiar with, to be able to recognise

    (i) the actual experienced quality of particular types of experience-contents, experience-constellations, and experience-sequences ;

    (ii) a class of object or objective entity or occurrence.

(2) To possess information, of any and every kind (correct representations and anticipations).

(3) To believe with complete assurance, on adequate grounds, and rightly.

(4) To confront in direct and immediate apprehension.

We may comment very briefly :

(13), (1) We have already acknowledged (i) as a basic psychological fact, in effect *the* most basic cognitive fact. But we have pointed out that (ii), though we also talk of it as acquaintance and recognition, is something quite different and vastly more sophisticated. It implies indeed a whole past history of learning ; the accumulation and organisation of information ; the presence in our minds of complex representation-patterns ; and the activation of these in expectation-form through a primary re-cognitive occurrence of the (i) type. In other words, meaning (1), (ii) is a telescoped combination of (1), (i) and (2).

(2) This covers the whole of what we normally call knowledge : science, history, memory, practical and personal information, etc. —We usually think of information as *about* some subject or other ; i.e., we presuppose that we are acquainted with different kinds of subjects (existents), and we talk of what we know about them (their properties, connections, interactions, relations, locations, durations, distributions, and so on). But this presupposed acquaintance is merely the counterpart once more of the acquaintance or recognition of our meaning (1), (ii), and can be shown to consist mainly or altogether of bodies of information. That is to say, of representations of linked and organised experience-contents, each element of which we are acquainted with and are able to recognise in sense (1), (i), whilst any encounter with a sufficient combination of these elements will cause us to recognise the presence of the whole. And even our knowledge of the *existence* of this or that class of subject is mainly or entirely a learnt complex of information, as our next section will show. It can indeed also be described as information *about* this or that part or domain of our total experience-world.

We have made use of the qualified term " mainly " because we do not need to assume in advance of our analysis that this will leave no unresolvable remainder ; the argument is merely that we must first allow fully for everything which can be *shown* to be experientially learnt and built up, *before* we start postulating primal or transcendental mysteries. It is just the potency of the learning process, when followed right through from the start in all its breadth and through all its cumulative history, that our philosophy has in the past missed, since only an adequate empirical psychology can supply it. What (if anything) is left over after the *complete* story of our experiential learning has been told is a question which must be deferred until then. The issue will, how-ever, be briefly referred to again below, in connection with meaning (4).

We should still note, in connection with (2), that the chief accent falls here on cognitive *content*, i.e., on the *possession* of infor-mation, as contrasted with its lack (or ignorance). The informa-tion is of course assumed to be true, i.e., to be in the main soundly established ; but when we use the term " knowledge " in this sense, we do not normally think of it as something absolutely rigorous and completely indubitable. In fact it is plain that the vast conglomerates of what we commonly so call (scientific, practical, personal, historical) must inevitably include, at any one time, quite an appreciable admixture of error. No sensible person would deny this—or on that account stop using the term knowledge for all our social stores of accepted information.

(3) The foregoing leads straight on to meaning (3), where, on the contrary, we focus specifically on the question of *valid assurance of truth*. Here the contrast is with error, on the one hand, and with " mere " belief or opinion, which may well be erroneous, on the other hand. This meaning of " knowing " is obviously a main rallying point of philosophic dispute. The issues of what are valid grounds for assurance, what are our ultimate grounds for assurance, and what the assurance is an assurance of, i.e. the meaning and criterion of truth, become tangled up with one another in the most inextricable way, and the result is an endless circular round of argument which in practice only adds up to deadlock.

For us the position is quite clear. Truth is correspondence of beliefs with objective facts (in the sense of " objective facts " which we have already partly defined and shall be defining further, and which gives a clear-cut experiential content to such correspondence). Knowledge consists of the beliefs of every kind for which we claim correspondence on generally dependable grounds. As most of them are continually being re-tested and re-confirmed, directly or indirectly, we can confidently maintain our assurance of truth, even whilst acknowledging that their sum probably contains some admixture of beliefs which close individual scrutiny might show to be doubtful or actually erroneous.

(14), (4) Meaning (4) is the central mystery of the philosophic theory of knowledge. It starts traditionally from the supposed confrontation of subject and object in perception or sensation, which, however, under critical fire soon loses, or appears to lose, its original semblance of directness and simplicity, and eventually breaks up into endless controversy and chaos. Nevertheless something, however difficult to define precisely, has always tended to survive ; some supposed implication of the act of knowing or of the fact of knowledge (or even of the very idea), according to which somehow, somewhere there is direct and immediate confrontation of a subject or knower with some sort of object or known and an ensuing direct and immediate apprehension of the latter—if only we could find out *what* it is that is thus so ultimately and indubitably " known."

Our empirical psychological approach postpones this mystery ; how much of it is left, or in what form, after our full factual survey is completed, is once more an open question. Meanwhile we are not here drawing at all on sense (4) of the terms " knowing " and " knowledge." We substitute for this sense the minimal subjective term " experiencing," which makes no such epistemological claim, i.e. which does not pretend to involve " knowing " in any sense, but merely provides the raw material for the further purely psychological processes of retention, recognition (sense of " like-something-before "), linkage of co-repeated experience-constellations, and revival with anticipation. But these processes, without any initial postulate of an original, more or less transcendental act of " knowing," can be shown to engender beliefs capable of truth or falsity and testable and tested for truth or falsity. Those beliefs which survive all such testing are our first knowledge. Certain of them, of particularly wide scope, allow us to build further and further on them and become the foundation for all the cumulative bodies of dependable information or knowledge which we gather throughout our individual and collective human history. And the most central and far-reaching and literally fundamental of these learnt beliefs, formed from the most impressive and enduring inter-relations and convergences of all our experiences, is precisely that which we describe as our belief in the existence of objects, objective happenings and the objective world. Our next section will deal in detail with its experiential basis and content.

Our use of the terms " knowing " and " knowledge " or " cognition " is thus based essentially on meaning (2), the possession of information (or, psychologically speaking, beliefs or representations with well-grounded assurance of truth). Our empirical psychological problem of knowledge is essentially how all our different kinds of mainly true information, and their eventual comprehensive systems, have been acquired. We interpret " information " in the broadest way, and do not *exclude the possibility* that some of this, perhaps even some ultimate core, may have been obtained by processes of direct apprehension or " knowing " in sense (4), or for that matter by various other means which have at different times been put forward. This will be discussed further in Chapter VIII. We claim only that we need not *start* with any such assumptions and can go an immensely long way towards covering all the traditional ground of our " knowledge," including most of its supposed central philosophic mysteries, by the simple method of an accurate and adequate and full description of the cumulative historical process of our familiar experiencing, and learning from experience. Accordingly we are suggesting that that should be carried through first, and only then should we consider what is left on our hands and what further suppositions or postulates this calls upon us to make.

CHAPTER IV

EXPERIENTIAL BASIS FOR OUR BELIEF IN THE OBJECTIVE WORLD (1)

I.—GENERAL SURVEY OF THE PROBLEM

(1) In order to provide a reasonably clear picture of what this section sets out to do, it may be useful to anticipate its detailed course by a certain amount of general discussion. This should, however, be regarded as purely elucidatory and without any claim other than to outline what is later on to be established.

(2) It must be emphasised first of all that we are only concerned here with the *experiential basis* for our belief in the existence of an objective world. This belief may go beyond that basis, or it may have roots that reach below it. We are not pronouncing on these questions. Our thesis is merely, here as all the way through, that before anything else we must start with a proper and adequate account of what our experience itself—the plain everyday pattern and biographical story of our own states—has to tell us. Our suggestion will be that this alone goes a remarkably long way not only towards explaining but towards justifying our ordinary " common sense " belief, or rather set of beliefs. We shall find that there is an immense system of separate but inter-supporting *learnt facts* about our perceptual experience which we can identify as entering into that set of beliefs and which together give us something extraordinarily like its familiar scheme. And by " learnt facts "—as has already been made clear—we do not mean more than actual experiential findings about the character of our perceptual experiences and their relationships to one another and to other kinds of experience ; but findings which achieve that status only because they have been continually tested and verified, combined, built upon, extended and re-verified, in a way which has put it almost beyond our power to question them. In effect, we shall suggest that the whole system of these " learnt facts " can be found and re-confirmed, independently of any theoretical assumptions or postulates, in our actual adult experience of any one day. We shall subsequently try to bring out some of the main learning processes of our earlier history by which the system is first built up. But the vital point is

that every day and all day long throughout our story we are
acting upon every element of it, in our special cognitive sense of
" acting upon," i.e., we are confronting our further experience
with an immense and close-knit scheme of expectations based upon
that system of learnt facts, and a vast pattern of prepared responses based in turn upon that expectation-scheme.   And the
further experience which moment by moment actually happens
must of necessity test, and does in fact always confirm that scheme
(in its main features, even if not in every detail).[1]

(3) That of course is why the ordinary person is so surprised
and bewildered when he first meets the traditional philosophic
battery of criticisms of his " naïve " common sense beliefs ; and
that is why, although he is quite unable to answer them and they
may well seem to him at first very convincing and very disturbing,
he is even more unable to *accept* them—or indeed, after the initial
impact, to take them really seriously.   He can in effect only deal
with them by regarding them as part and parcel of some peculiar
philosophers' world, which is their affair and not his, and on
which, half in real, half in mock humility, he turns his back,
whilst for his own part he goes on his accustomed way.

But for exactly the same reasons the philosopher himself, however seriously he thinks he is taking his doubts and with whatever
conviction he works out his own alternative (which may seem to
be something utterly different from the naïve common sense world),
continues to act on precisely the same set of beliefs as he did prior
to his doubts and to his alternative *true* view, and as does the
ordinary person.   He cannot alter the too firmly learnt history
which is acting in him, he cannot fly in the face of what he *knows*
to be the facts (a myriad connected ones ;   all the far-flung
system of *detailed* findings which we mean by our belief in the
common sense world).   Unless he goes quite literally mad, he will
not even *try* to alter any part of this common sense scheme of
beliefs in his practice ;   to do so is in effect to become incapable of
looking after oneself and certifiably insane.   Neither can one
treat the scheme as in real doubt, i.e., seek to suspend it, without
returning to something like the state of complete helplessness and
intellectual vacuity of the new-born child.   Practically everything
which the grown-up person can *successfully* do, from the smallest
adjustment to the largest planned activity, practically everything

---

[1] It is important to note that, whenever a particular expectation is falsified, the
main containing scheme is, at one and the same time, always *verified*, so that it actually
gains in overall strength by each of these limited local breakdowns.

which differentiates the structure of his experience and behaviour from that of the new-born infant, rests upon just that scheme of beliefs.

(4) If then we can show that there is a system of learnt experiential " facts," or tested and verified experiential beliefs, which constitutes at the least a large part of our affirmation of an objective world, we shall no doubt still be left with the question whether there is anything more in this belief that is not so accounted for. If there is, it may be a matter for philosophic consideration, though even so, there may yet be a prior psychological problem for factual inquiry.[1] But in any event we shall hope to establish that what is open to question and discussion is, by comparison, only a marginal element, and that we stultify our thinking in advance if, in the customary philosophic fashion, we plunge straight into dialectical debate *pro* and *contra* our belief in the objective world, without ascertaining the full and verifiable psychological picture first.

(5) Before, however, we proceed to our more detailed psychological description, there is a challenge which it seems desirable, even if only in a preliminary way, to try to meet. It may be pointed out that our so-called common sense beliefs are nothing so clear-cut or homogeneous as the present approach would appear to postulate. They are obviously very vague and fluctuating, they vary widely at different times even in the same person, they can be shown to involve elements of manifest self-contradiction, etc., etc.

We might answer by referring the reader to our actual description, which will bring out concretely just what set of beliefs is meant here ; whilst any advance discussion in general terms must tend to involve us in just that premature philosophising which we are seeking to avoid. Nevertheless, it is true that there are certain difficulties and certain qualifying factors which are best acknowledged at the start, and our enterprise can only be helped by a general clearing of the air, so long as it remains understood that this is mere preparation for the strictly psychological account to follow.

(i) There are undoubtedly wide variations between the " common sense " world-pictures of people of different levels of education, of laymen and of scientists, and of young children and adults even in the same social group ; there is a very large margin of vagueness about the world-map of the non-scientific public ;

[1] See Chapter VIII below.

and there are definite clashes between the ordinary " common sense " and the strictly scientific pictures. But it is possible never-theless to sort out this seemingly heterogeneous material into two main groupings ; to indicate broadly the clash between them ; and to show that after all it does not penetrate as deeply as may at first appear and that underneath it there is a large core of agreement which can legitimately be referred to as the (firmly validated) common sense belief in the existence of the objective world, in the very way in which we have done.

(ii) The starting point of the common sense set of beliefs is of course the naïve assumption of the veridicity of perception. The latter is held to give us direct access to a world of things outside us, which we apprehend through seeing, hearing, touching, etc., just as in fact they are. Thus perception is supposed to disclose to us the existence and character of objects and objective entities in the spatial world around us (i.e. around our bodies, which are them-selves similar even if very special objects in space), and also the occurrence of all sorts of events and proceedings in that same spa-tial world. By a further extension of the same processes we take in the fact that these objects, etc., follow their own courses, inde-pendently of us and of whether we happen to be paying attention to them or not, and have their own past, equally independently of whether we were there to witness it or not. By the same token we go on to appreciate that if we do suitably pay attention to these objects and their courses, whilst at the same time we make full use of what we have already learnt about them, we can con-tinue to find out more and more about them, alike as regards their present, their future and their past.

(iii) The *basic* common sense set of beliefs we have just outlined leaves room obviously for the most widely varying views about what there is in the objective world besides the familiar objects and occurrences of our everyday perception, and what the relationship is between the latter and any realities which we do not apprehend in that straightforward, self-evident way. There are, on every showing, very many facts (experiences) to complicate and blur to some extent any over-simple picture of perceived material objects and well-defined, concrete, physical events. But we are only concerned here with the truth that whatever *further* beliefs the ordinary common sensible member of our society may entertain, he does carry along with him the assumption of the reality, more or less as he perceives it, of all his surrounding " object " world of tables and chairs and domestic appliances, houses and towns, vehicles and machines, trees and other plants, animals and his fellow men, together with their relations and inter-actions with one another, and their own past and future. And of course with the fully retained belief in this world of objects and events there goes an equal assurance about the similarly perceived material and objective world of their setting : fields and rivers, plains and mountains and valleys, lakes and oceans, continents and our whole earth (as itself an object in a larger space).

(6), (iv) On the other hand, however, there are two orders of facts which impinge directly on this set of beliefs and introduce qualifications, disparities and perplexities into it. The first con-sists of everything that happens even within our ordinary ex-perience which throws doubt on the assumed simple veridicity of perception. The second arises from the gradual development of our scientific world-picture, i.e., the picture science has worked out of what " really " underlies the world of our apparent sensible objects and their seeming interactions and vicissitudes.

The first order of facts provides the initial stimulus and material for philosophic questioning, challenges and speculations. Optical illusions and deflections, mirages, hallucinations, dreams, and all the familiar relativities of perception are common occurrences, which no one can altogether overlook. But the ordinary person, without any special predisposition towards the interests and attitudes we call philosophic, comes to rough-and-ready terms with these experiences and goes his way : he distinguishes between semblance and reality, segregates dreams and pathological con-ditions, allows for a margin of errors, aberrations and distortions, but still holds on to his main belief in the veridicity of careful and confirmed perception under satisfactory conditions, and *pari passu* in the reality *and so-ness* of the world with which this perception acquaints him.

The second order of facts is less easily dealt with and all that the ordinary educated person can do about it is to cleave to his common sense world, because he cannot dispense with it, but at the same time to try to assimilate and accept what he can grasp of the scientific world-picture, in its many different aspects. What the relation is between the two, and even between different parts of the scientific world-picture itself, is not his worry. He is aware, moreover, that during the past few decades the basic scientific picture has greatly changed, that it is still in large part under fundamental debate among scientists themselves and that in any event much of it has moved on to a plane of abstruseness and mathematical intricacy which he cannot hope to follow. Nevertheless, to reassure himself a little, he can tell himself that neither the macrocosmic astronomical pattern nor the microcosmic chemical one with which he had become familiar have lost their previous main shape : from the sun and planets and the larger stellar universe at the one extreme, to the various elemental atoms which behave in so many ways just like ordinary perceptual unit-objects, and (he is assured) can even be " split " by being " bombarded " with smaller and more ultimate particles, at the other extreme. And at least the proximate astronomical pattern given by those essentially scientific instruments, the telescope and the camera, has every appearance of being just an expansion and enlargement of our ordinary perceptual picture. Therefore the average educated person believes concurrently in the common sense perceptual world and in what he can understand of the macrocosmic and microcosmic scientific world, whilst leaving it to whomever it may concern to work out their bearings on one another and in particular those of the world depicted by science on the common sense assumption of the simple veridicity of perception.

As for the more directly disruptive impact on this assumption of all the work done on the physiology of the nerve system and of the sense organs, the ordinary layman is hardly aware of any problem. He cannot indeed avoid taking note of the fact, which is apt to obtrude itself from time to time, that perception depends not only on the existence but also on the specific character and structure of his sense organs, and is liable to be affected by every variation of these. But he draws no further conclusions from these occasional findings in particular instances, and maintains his common sense world-picture, together with the assumptions on which it is based, exactly as before. The philosopher who follows up these cases soon becomes involved in an inextricable tangle of difficulties not merely over the physiological conditions and limitations of perception but also over the very status of these physiological facts once perception is thus subjectivised ; whilst quite apart from that radical perplexity, even the mutual compatibility of the nerve-physiological scientific picture and the physical one is not clear. But the ordinary person finds that he need pay no more attention to these later complications (if he comes across them) than to their starting points in his own familiar experience : the important point is that with only minor local qualifications and adjustments he can go on undisturbedly treating his common sense assumptions as correct. And of course it is also true that, as we have already remarked, for all practical purposes the philosopher does the same.

(v) If the foregoing is a just sketch of the current state of affairs, we must think of two main forms of belief in an objective physical world, which are held conjointly by contemporary common sense, though one in a much more vague and incomplete form than the other : belief in the perceived sensible order of things, and belief in the world, or worlds, of science. There is a clash, or an apparent clash, between them, because the former assumes the general veridicity of perception, whilst the latter seems largely to undermine and reject this. Scientists, obviously, take their stand on the second picture, but it must be noted that in practice they too continue to work on our naïve perceptual assumptions, just like the philosophers who formally challenge these and so often and cogently disprove them.

We have here a situation which seems in many ways paradoxical. For most philosophers indeed the clinging of virtually everybody, including even themselves, in their daily life, to the naïve perceptual world-model offers no particular difficulty : they regard this as just a primitive metaphysics which has become a habit and can be clung to because it is only idle theory that normally makes no difference. And if they still adhere to the habit themselves, that is only like still talking, or even thinking, of the sun rising and setting and moving round the earth. We shall, however, offer precisely the opposite explanation. We shall suggest that on the contrary the naïve perceptual world-picture is clung to because, in spite of all apparent difficulties, on the whole it works ; because indeed it is the only one that will work ; and because most of its content is in fact continually re-tested and re-confirmed, so that it cannot be disbelieved. That is why ordinary people can afford to disregard those difficulties, and not merely so, but must disregard them ; and why scientists and philosophers behave in practice just like ordinary people, whatever seemingly incompatible views they may in theory profess.

(7), (vi) For the solution of the paradox, at any rate as between the ordinary person and the scientist, we may first emphasise again that they are not really as far apart as a too antithetical mode of statement can make them appear. The scientific view of the world, in its different aspects, has *developed continuously* out of the naïve perceptual one, still leans on this, and retains a number of fundamental features in common with it. We are still local and temporary objects or object-histories surrounded in space and time by a far larger world which is mainly independent, in existence and activity and history, of our existence and history, and above all independent of the happening or not-happening of the acts by which we take fragmentary cognisance of it. In these respects the scientific picture has merely extended a myriad-fold the scale in time and space of our naïve objective world.

Secondly, the naïve assumption of the simple and direct veridicity or revelatoriness of perception must no doubt go, but the whole secret of the extraordinary growth of knowledge under the aegis of scientific method is that it not only retains but underlines, more than had ever been done before, the status and authority of perception which went with that naïve assumption. And though we cannot defend our initial belief that perception directly declares to us the nature of objects and occurrences exactly as they are, by and large we must behave as if it did. Why? Because it continues to operate as a true key—and our main if not perhaps our only key—to an order of things independent of us and controlling us *which we have to acknowledge.* Because this applies point by point in such wise that we have to acknowledge a controlling order of objective entities and occurrences somehow equivalent in practically every detail to what our perceptual experience delivers to us. And because so far from this being mere idle theory, it is forced upon us by the entire natural history of our perceptual experience in among all the rest of our states. In effect that particular kind of psychic happening (only marked out to begin with by its specific recognitive characters or set of felt qualities) segregates itself more and more from the rest, as it gathers round itself a great connected system of distinguishing coefficients. And these, we find, give it a unique status as that element in our total experience which *stands for* the objective reality that controls its main course.

(vii) We shall be developing this theme fully in our detailed psychological description. The point to note here is that the unbreakable link between our naïve common sense world-picture and our subsequent scientific one is the special dominant status of our perceptual experience. For the one as for the other, this remains the direct vehicle between ourselves and the world of fact and reality surrounding us. We have already brought out some of the central features of that status when in our previous chapter we exhibited perceptual experience as first, the chief *source* of our beliefs (i.e., our cumulative information), secondly the stimulus which from case to case activates the relevant ones (as expectations), and thirdly and above all as the running test of truth or falsity of these beliefs. It is in this last guise that it stands out most clearly as the principle of fact-control on which all scientific method is ultimately based.

In the broadest terms, primary perceptual experience is the mode of experience which comes to us as the *actual fact* (involuntary, obligatory, extraneous—that which has to be acknowledged) as distinct from our own previous state, or all that we merely think or believe, wish or fear.[1]

(8) It may be pointed out here against us that if it is an advantage, it is also a severe limitation that all that can ever happen on our view, in so-called fact-control, is that actual primary experience of the perceptual kind verifies (or falsifies) previous representations of such experience, based on past experienced concurrences. In other words, the whole process remains incurably inside our own states ; our view is condemned to stay to the end as phenomenalist or subjectivist as it was at the beginning, and the suggestion that if only we start from a complete enough subjectivism, we shall transcend this from within, stands self-refuted.

But of course we have so far only brought in a fraction of the story, and the remainder is just what this and the next chapter are intended to supply. For the moment we are only concerned to emphasise that whatever science, i.e. scientific method, may ultimately tell us about the nature of our physical world, this

---

[1] There is a range of exceptions to the rule of fact-control through primary perceptual experience, but it is of the kind that proves its rule. We have in effect, in our previous chapter, spoken of primary experience generally, and not only of the perceptual class, as the supervening order of facts which tests our beliefs ; though we have stressed that the perceptual order is far and away the main one. The exceptions consist of course of the beliefs and expectations which we should call psychological in the specialised sense, i.e., those which refer to our *merely* subjective or personal states —such as pains and pleasures or feelings of any kind. These modes of primary experience, when they actually happen, either correspond or fail to correspond with what we were forepicturing, that is, they verify or falsify these anticipations or beliefs, in exactly the same way as an actual perception may verify or falsify an expected one. And everybody will agree that the notion of fact is as applicable to the actual occurrence of personal feeling states as to any other sort of event, and stands in just the same relation to our advance beliefs about these states.

Thus the principle of fact-control in psychology, in contrast to all other sciences, does *not* call automatically for control by primary perceptual experience, but is satisfied by the confrontation of our psychological beliefs with whatever form of primary experiencing they may happen to refer to. But even so it remains significantly true that the work of scientific psychological inquiry and the establishment of stable psychological truth are vastly facilitated if tests, even though indirect, by primary perceptual experience can be introduced. There is great methodological merit in the principle of behaviourism, if only it is interpreted widely (humanly and historically) enough.

cannot but be compatible with the acceptance of the controlling status of perception as the key to that world, since the ultimate test is always agreement of the theory with the facts of observation and experiment (or rather, the observed outcome of experiment). Primary perceptual experience thus fully retains its place as final arbiter, as it were for and on behalf of the objective world.

And it is also desirable to stress here in advance that on the present view the propositions about the objective world which are thus brought to the test are *not* merely beliefs about actual or possible perceptual experience. They are beliefs which in the last resort can only be tested through such experience ; but they are about things which exist or have existed independently of us and apart from us, at least in the sense in which we ourselves exist ; or about things which are happening or will happen or have happened independently of us and apart from us, at least in the sense in which things are happening or will happen or have happened in our own history. This true content of our beliefs is made particularly plain by all those about the past, where there can be no question now of actual experience, and where nothing is further from our minds than any notion of the dependence of what we believe on a human being chancing to be there to witness it (e.g., the formation of the first igneous rocks, or the birth of a star). We must be ready to recognise, as soon as we carefully consider the psychological history and contents of our ideas, that we can believe nothing and describe nothing except in terms ultimately of actual experience of ours (however much imaginatively extended and enlarged) ; we must also be ready to recognise that we have little reason to suppose that these give us the nature of things as they actually are. We must therefore acknowledge that any statement we make about past existences or occurrences, even as about distant ones, is always a statement in terms of what we should have experienced (witnessed or observed) if we had been there—and had had all the opportunities and capacities needed to take in the particular nature and scale of the occurrence we were postulating. Yet behind this acknowledgment there is always the belief that what we perceptually observe or witness bears a direct relationship to what is there and happening, and stands for it feature by feature, event by event, point by point. Perceptual experience does not " represent " objective actuality in the sense of picturing or mirroring it, but it is representative of this in the sense that (in so far as it is carefully controlled and checked), it carries throughout its own course the stamp and authority of objective actuality and provides at least a true and faithful *counterpart* to it.

(9) All this must now be left to be filled in by the present and the following two chapters. It is important to register that these require to be read together : the beliefs in objective existence and in causality, or causal control, are complementary parts of a single integral whole. The notion of control will in effect play a crucial role even in the present section. It is merely for practical convenience that we are focusing attention first of all on that grouping of experiences which is expressed most naturally as the belief in the existence of an objective world, and then separately on that grouping of largely the same set of experiences which is brought together in our belief in causality.

We shall seek to show in this and the following chapter how every feature which is *shared* by the common sense and the scientific picture of the objective world (and we have already indicated that what is thus shared is in fact the main substance of both) appears as an actual class of experiences that is continually re-encountered and re-confirmed and becomes combined with the rest in a single organic system of learnt facts or truths-of-experience. It is this system of verified truths-of-experience which common sense affirms and clings to when it stands by its belief in the objective world and (quite rightly) rejects, as somehow irrelevant, even the most plausible argument against that belief.

(10) Before we go on to our outline of the system (at first taken cross-sectionally, then genetically), there is one point already touched upon which it may be useful to expand a little.

As we have indicated, the child's first picture of the objective world falls naturally into three related but separable parts. There is first the background field, the more or less constant and immobile arena of his perceptual experience to which he pays only limited attention but which nevertheless gradually registers in his memory as a framework, varying as he himself is moved about but hardly otherwise. There are secondly, and most importantly, an ever growing number of single, discrete, mobile objects, of every sort of size, character and behaviour : toys, utensils, articles of food, humans, animals, etc. And thirdly there are events and processes, from regular routines to every kind of irruptive novelty —most often involving objects and consisting of happenings to them or things being done to or by them.

We have noted that of these three orders of objective actuality, the second becomes in many ways the most typical for the child's belief in a world outside him ; that is, in a world of entities existing independently of him and having a reality and life and history of their own just as he has. Objects give him the most varied and most exciting and important experiences and provide the easiest cases from which to learn the lesson of the objective world. The more constant and immobile features of the world round him tend merely to appear as a stage on which these real entities live and move and have their being. Whilst happenings and events are in the main just their dramatic doings and under-goings.

But gradually the other two orders of actuality get expanded in their turn ; the world of discrete object-entities loses some of its simplicity, all sorts of intermediate or combined cases turn up, and everything becomes intertwined and fused in one single objective order. The child detaches some portions of the pre-vious *framework* and sees them as after all themselves single, dis-crete and movable if not very mobile objects. He takes in a larger and still larger framework, in the light of which his whole previous one becomes a single object. He learns to recognise groups and assemblages of things as connected wholes. He becomes familiar with substances which are not discrete single entities, and also with more and more complex courses of events, with processes and situations, with occasions, relations, properties, etc. He comes furthermore to see that there are substances which are not even usually perceptible (air, gas, etc.). And so on. In many such experiences some of the most obvious coefficients of objectivity of those easy instances, single discrete mobile objects, are lacking. But firstly, they still share so many of the distinctive characters of the latter and secondly, they are so continuous with them, that it is clear that our only course is to widen and widen the notion of objective existence and occurrence till it embraces all of them. In the end it covers anything and everything which exists or occurs (and can be recognised or identified) in the spatial field outside the individual's body—and of course also everything that exists or occurs within that body as itself an occupant of the same spatial field.

Eventually the wider extensions of that field virtually swamp the child's original ego-centric collection of objects, which are found to throw only a very limited light on the character and structure of the objective world as a whole. Yet on the other hand, as we have seen, the notion of object, in the original sense of a single, discrete, mobile entity having its own characteristic place

c

and properties in the space outside him, retains much of its central importance. Beneath un-object-like substances like water or gases, there appear object-like entities such as molecules and atoms ; and even when these yield to further breaking down, we get more ultimate entities which still seem to have enough in common with single, discrete, mobile objects to be describable (at least in some of their aspects) as distinct particles, i.e., as neutrons, electrons, etc., capable of being separated and combined, of being used as projectiles, of being captured and escaping, and so on.[1]

Moreover, our very objects of everyday life retain a more distinctive status than we often give them credit for ; thus for the scientist even more than for the ordinary person, the *boundaries* of a penny lying on a table are the *boundaries* of a wholly different set of controlling constituents, characteristics, properties and relationships from those of the table under the penny, and the air round it. And so with every familiar object around us. We may repeat that in effect perception *maintains* what we may call a *virtual veridicity*, which we have to continue to acknowledge, and to be guided by at all times. The degree to which the most advanced scientists not only take for granted but rely upon the objective just-so-ness of typical ordinary perceptual objects can be illustrated in innumerable further ways. We need only consider for example their dependence upon this just-so-ness in regard to all their laboratory utensils, vessels and equipment and above all their scientific instruments of every kind. And the same applies obviously also to such starting points or subject-matters of their

---

[1] Since I am not a physicist, I am conscious of the imprudence of the above plunge into matters beyond my depth. It has often been insisted that the authentic teaching of physics is embodied in mathematical statements which are incapable of translation into ordinary language. For the purposes of popular exposition, rough metaphors and analogies have to be introduced, but must not on any account be taken literally, and indeed though some properties of the terms of our equations lend themselves to the analogy of particles, others just as plainly do not and suggest the altogether different notion of waves. And so forth.

Like other laymen I can but accept this, as far as I am able to understand it, whilst appreciating that the mathematical true inwardness of present-day physical-chemical doctrine must escape me. But I do suggest that it is also relevant that as soon as physicists themselves go outside their strict mathematical context and apply it, whether in language or in action, to the actual world of phenomena, they become involved in far more psychology (of knowledge) than they themselves are aware of. It would not be difficult to show how readily—and how unconsciously—they in turn move out of their depth. In this connection attention might usefully be focused, for a start, on the very convenient but very uncritical common use by scientists of the notion of convenience. But these complicated matters cannot be thrashed out here.—I must be content if my brief trespasses into the physical field are free from gross errors ; and in this modest purpose I have been guided by numerous authoritative scientific pronouncements and hope therefore I have not failed.

work as pieces of mineral or rock or, with only very minor modifications, quantities of powders or liquids in test tubes or bottles or on microscope slides. The case of the botanist and zoologist and biologist generally is, if anything, more obvious still. The scientist assumes the common sense world more continuously, comprehensively and deliberately than anyone else.

In the following very summary exposé we shall find it convenient to focus much of our psychological description of the experience-sources and experience-contents of our belief in the objective world on the easy and simple case of concrete objects. Hence the desirability of bringing out their pervasive and sustained significance, plus the existence of a ready and adequate passage from them to every other constituent of our world. And whilst, for the limited purposes of the present prefatory section, we have allowed ourselves the free use of " object language " even before we have justified this psychologically, it may perhaps already be apparent how little any full account of our experience as such can do without all the detailed distinctions and acknowledgments embodied in that language.

II.—PRELIMINARY CROSS-SECTIONAL APPROACH TO COMMON SENSE
ADULT BELIEF

(11) If we now turn to our actual phenomenological description, there are good reasons—as will, I think, be seen—for starting with a preliminary cross-sectional approach, but it will be apparent that this must cover substantially the same ground as our proposed genetic picture. To minimise repetition, therefore, the former will be confined here to a bare sketch, intended chiefly to serve as a frame of reference and means of check of the genetic story.

We can set out from almost any experiential state, such as my sitting at my typewriter in my study, and consider what I am actually experiencing (i.e. in the primary mode) ; what, over and above this, I am believing ; and why. But there is perhaps a special fitness in our choosing for our starting point a state such as waking up from a night's sleep and for a moment taking in *newly* where we are and what is happening to us, against the very sense of previous blankness.

We become aware then more or less concurrently of several components in our state : chiefly of a perceptual one (itself complex, though most prominent as a varied visual field), but usually also of diverse other elements : perhaps a feeling of sleepiness, perhaps one of euphoria ; possibly a craving as of hunger ; perhaps also a sudden recollection of something that happened or that we thought of last night ; perhaps a recurring image from a dream ; possibly an anticipation of something about to happen in a moment (e.g., somebody going to bring a cup of tea), or a surge of determination to get up quickly this morning.

Several of these components may be present together, but the perceptual and above all the visual-perceptual one will stand out with a characteristic quality, or set of qualities, of its own. (i) It has the visuo-kinaesthetic characters of a spatial field : continuity ; a focal structure ; the possibility of shifting the focus whilst retaining a large part of the previous field ; that of maintaining a given focus more or less indefinitely ; and that of relinquishing and recovering a given focus more or less indefinitely. (ii) It carries with it a special, distinctive coefficient of attitude and activity on our part : attention, or ad-tension, a directed receptiveness, capable (*a*) of staying put, (*b*) of following, and (*c*) of itself taking the lead, always with the same quality of tautness, but waiting tautness, tautness ready to take in. (iii) And the perceptual state also carries with it, in peculiarly intimate fusion, a whole set of beliefs which we can indeed separate out of that fusion, and some of which are at times forcibly *proved* separate through being shown false, but which for the most part appear to us to be part of the immediate perceptual content itself.

(12) These beliefs include, most strictly speaking, those rudimentary ones which we have referred to as the very characters of the field itself : the *possibilities* of maintaining, shifting and recovering particular foci which go beyond the immediate present, however imperceptibly they *grow* out of this. But more substantially the beliefs in question consist of all those summed up in the assumption that we are looking into a spatial field outside ourselves and independent of ourselves, and within that field are looking at a grouping of separate, independent objects and (if our perceptual content changes as we keep our attention steady and remain watching) objective or " real " events. Thus the visual-perceptual content of our total state appears to *present* itself to us with the character of a seeing of a table and chairs, a glass and a vase with flowers, etc., etc., which are really " there " outside us. And, if we are looking at a window, we are seeing the actual happening " there " of a fly walking up and down the pane, or, if looking at the door, we are watching its actual opening and somebody coming in with a tray and a cup of tea.

However, this apparently single assumption that the visual-perceptual component in our total state is a seeing of real objects and events can quite easily, as it were by mere shaking up or stirring, be made to translate itself into a whole series of distinct but connected beliefs going beyond the immediately present experience-content. The latter is not merely something imagined or remembered or felt or desired but, quite differently from all these states of our own selves, is regarded as an apprehension of things really there and of events really happening in and among them. What makes us think that? What do we mean by it? How do we know it or are we sure of it? Why, because our state is one of directed attention held and controlled by something outside itself (whether passively fixed upon it, actively and mobilely exploring it, or, again passively, following it). Because, in so far as we are looking at something which we recognise as an *object*, we believe, on the strength of our entire past experience, that (i) we can move towards it (towards the visual shape) ; (ii) we can develop the visual shape further ; (iii) we can complete it by touching it and manually exploring it and tracing its contours ; (iv) we can (in the typical case of a not too large solid object) detach the visual-tactile shape from its setting and move it (lift it or shift it) as a single whole ; (v) we can act upon it and change it ; (vi) we can frequently use it to change other such objects ; (vii) we can foresee the character of these various changes before they are brought about ; (viii) we can tell from the state of this or that object that such and such changes have already occurred in it, and we can then find further perceptual facts also pointing to such changes ; (ix) by attentional-perceptual focusing either on a particular object or on others like it and watching their course we can learn more and more about their whole class ; (x) by a wide range of exploratory actions on and with these objects, combined with attentional-perceptual focusing, we can further greatly increase our learnt knowledge about them ; (xi) but from time to time they will falsify this apparent knowledge and compel us to attend to them anew and to learn better about them. And so on. In so far as we are watching *happenings*, we can locate them in and among objects, we can relate them to these in the various ways we have just described, and we are in fact throughout building up information about them at the same time as about objects. And *all these are actual distinctive experiences* which we do in fact get anew the whole time.

(13) Not every one of the foregoing characteristics will be applicable to every object, but in the case of many of them there will be a good many more, and anyway there will be continuity and large overlaps between them and they will all appear as members of the same context or order or " objective " world. And what we shall say and feel is that these are *some* of the characteristics we mean when we affirm that we are seeing (touching, etc.) *real* objects, but that they are far from being exhaustive, and that the important point about them is that they are no mere series of separate and independent facts. They are closely linked together ; they support and develop one another ; and they conjointly confirm and indeed enforce the acknowledgment of (thus perceived) " real " objects—which then further demonstrate their reality (and that of the objective order of which they form part) in endless other ways.

Thus the case is *not* simply one of visual experiences being signs of the possibility of certain others, or even of groups of them. What we actually find is a *convergence of different types of experience*, each of them generating a characteristic kind of belief or expectation which carries with it something of the quality of the belief in objective thereness (from the initial conjunction of perception with attentional activity onward) ;. and all those different kinds fit in with one another and amalgamate into a single belief of which they form mutually consistent parts or facets. And of course this happens only because each of the components is in fact continually borne out and is thus built up further, both directly and in combination with the others. When on waking up in the morning we find as part of our total state the visual-perceptual content which we *recognise* as the familiar room round us, the table beside the bed, the window opposite, the glass and the watch on the table, etc., etc., it is obvious that hardly anything of all this is given to us even visually ; almost everything is *read into* our actual immediate experiential content (however intimately and interpenetratingly) and is at that first moment mere assumption and belief. But every aspect of the belief is successively confirmed. Our attention rests on a given area or object, and this remains " there " and the same, as long as we care to watch. Our glance moves away, and one thing after another, just as we are expecting it, comes into sight (if, very occasionally, something does not, we jump, and investigate). Our attention wanders back and we recover what we began with. We stretch out our hand towards the visual glass and, as we believed, it is a " real " glass, i.e., one which we can also lift up and move towards us and drink from—or carelessly push over the side of the table and shatter. We feel dry, and drink in order to be refreshed—and duly are so. Or the glass contains some medicine which we know to be disagreeable, and it does not fail us. And we can get up out of the " real " bed, on to the " real " floor and walk over to the " real " window, and open it, or open it wider. In fact we proceed about our usual morning routine in all its complexity of endless successive perceptions, expectations, actions, further expectations and perceptions. Every instant brings the anticipated further development of our experiences in their different but mutually dependent kinds. Everything happens in full accordance with our scheme of beliefs, and the latter is wholly pivoted on the assumption of an objective order which (*a*) we are perceiving and which (*b*) controls our course through the cue of our successive perceptions ; that is to say, to which we are adjusting ourselves continuously under the guidance of these perceptions.

(14) All this is however still only a minute fragment of our experience-course even of a single day. And we have not so far considered more than a fraction of its content. In particular, what is present in it equally is the set of perceptual contents which I refer to an object like any other, but somehow peculiarly and uniquely bound up with the entire course of my experiences : my body. This adds its own characteristic and constant contribution to our acknowledgment of all the various *other* objects we find to be similar in many ways, but separate and independent co-occupants of the same spatial field. That contribution is then in turn strengthened and consolidated by the way in which perception ushers in (mostly at an early stage of our morning scene) one or more objects extremely similar to our own bodily selves and believed, and verified as fast as believed, to be bound up with experiences parallel to our own. So parallel indeed that we can use theirs as if they were our own, and they in the same way ours, for the purpose of filling gaps in our own perception or in theirs.

But our early morning scene changes continuously into a series of others, all repeating the same underlying pattern, whilst at the same time introducing the most diverse new variations, and extending and enlarging the main theme in every direction. After breakfasting successfully (on the basis of innumerable further fulfilled assumptions about the " thereness " and " so-ness " of hosts of things) we proceed to our place of work and settle down to the latter, through an immense network of further confirmed expectations and beliefs. These, whether specific or general, are all of the same broad type as those of the first few minutes of our re-entry into our world after waking up. A great many are re-verified each instant as we go along, with every new movement of the eyes or hand, every turn of the head which shifts our perceptual field, every step we take and every form of practical adaptation or purposive action we carry out. And besides such habitual minor adjustments, most of us also bring to bear each day instalments of much more far-reaching schemes of planned behaviour which involve great organised systems of belief and assumption about the same objective world ; and these again are borne out in most of their detail as we proceed.

In effect, a day's life of any ordinary member of our society involves vast tracts of individual and social (communicated) information regarding our world—geographical, technological, economic, sociological, historical, etc.—and tests and confirms this at a myriad points and in a myriad ways. We can best realise the immense amount of massive, cumulative confirmation which we thus receive when it does happen that something goes awry, and mostly in trivial but occasionally in more important respects our assumptions or beliefs let us down. We are then more than ever, as we have seen, confronted with the objectivity of our objective world, but after the first jar it most often becomes clear that this is only a local and momentary failure of our expectation-scheme, which leaves all its main structure intact. And even in the few more serious cases we find that the basic structure fully survives and we merely have to reconstruct a limited local area. Whilst, most significantly of all, we have to reconstruct it in terms of that basic structure, i.e. in terms of further and better learning (attending, exploring, testing) of the real order of things, which is there and can only be coped with, in the interest of our own desires and needs, in so far as we learn *truly* to know it.

(15) Summarising our rapid cross-sectional sketch and at the same time providing a table of contents for the genetic outline to follow, we may say in generalised terms that our belief in our objective world rests upon—and as a minimum signifies—the *convergence and integration* of all the following main features of our experience, passive and active :

    (i) The focus-field character and field-continuity of perception.

(ii) The intimate, mutually controlling relationship between our perceptual experiences and our attentional activities (i.e. the experiences we designate as such).

(iii) The similar but further-reaching relationship of mutual control between our perceptual experiences and our locomotive activities (again, the experiences we designate as such).

(iv) The partly similar but partly different relationship of mutual control between our perceptual experiences and all our operative activities.

(v) The experienced dependence of our affective-conative course—obtainment and retention of the feeling-states we desire, relief from and avoidance of those we want to reject—on the presence, absence and variations of specific perceptual foci.

(vi) The possibility of anticipating correctly from a given perceptual experience, or a given attentional, locomotive or operative activity, the further course of our perceptual experience—but the possibility also that this anticipation may be falsified from time to time by the actual further course of perception.

(vii) The possibility of learning, by suitable new attentional activities, how to avoid particular falsified anticipations for the future.

(viii) The recognition of certain perceptual foci, i.e. those we call our own bodies, as standing in a unique controlling relation to *all* our experiences, but as nevertheless similar in many ways to most others (of the " object " type), and in most ways to many others—and so of these others as similar to the first.

(ix) The finding that all these other perceptual foci (of the object type) have futures and pasts of *their* own, just like our own.

(x) The recognition of the most similar class of these other perceptual foci as standing in the same relation to other selves, with experiences and experience-histories like our own, as the perceptual foci we call our own bodies stand to our own experiencing selves and our experience-history.

(xi) The possibility of interchanging not only present and past experiences but also anticipations of future experiences with these other bodily-psychic selves, in such a way that we can act successfully (at most times) on their anticipations, and they on ours.

(xii) The possibility and the rewards of an attitude of belief that there *is* an objective world of which, by the right combination of attentional activities (in all their most developed modes) and perceptual receptivity, we can learn to know more and more. A world which thereby we can learn to represent, in past, present and future, more and more *truly* and *fully*. And a world to which therefore we are able to adjust all our other activities (locomotive and operative) with more and more of the affective-conative success we are seeking.

All the foregoing features and factors of our past experience have together shaped the set of general assumptions and beliefs, and the behaviour informed and controlled by these, with which, moment by moment, we confront our further experience ; and it cannot be too much emphasised that the latter incessantly confirms all the main tenor of that set of beliefs. That is why we go on entertaining it, and why if challenged we must re-affirm it and can do no other. And we are simply registering the history and outcome of all our experience when we sum up that entire far-flung system of beliefs in the single *acknowledgment* of an objective world of endless diverse things and happenings in which our bodies are objects like any others ; in which we have our own place and biography as local parts of a vastly larger history ; and in which our particular story includes a progressive but always fractional learning-to-know about both itself and the rest.

CHAPTER V

EXPERIENTIAL BASIS FOR OUR BELIEF IN THE OBJECTIVE WORLD (2)

I.—GENETIC APPROACH : A PRELIMINARY DIFFICULTY

(1) From the foregoing cross-sectional approach to our organised adult experience we may now pass on to the slow-motion picture which our actual early history provides of the stages and processes by which we build up that organisation. We cannot indeed attempt more here than to sketch in the most summary way the rudimentary groundwork of this story ; a really adequate study would be a matter for volumes. That is brought out by the great mass of material in the standard works on early psychological development, which nevertheless, because of the nature of their assumptions, take much of the inner story for granted. It is not possible to cover their ground here, but what follows may perhaps be regarded as an introduction and key to the interpretation of their data from within.

However, this is not such a simple undertaking : there is a preliminary difficulty to be dealt with (which constitutes part of the reason why we began with our cross-sectional survey). It is obvious that any genetic reconstruction of what happens by way of organisation of our experience during our first two or three years must draw most of its supporting evidence from behaviouristic facts. Direct introspection can help us little if at all, nor can we get much aid from what we should usually describe as introspective evidence from others, i.e. their own report of their states, since children of less than say three have only the most limited range of articulate expression, and infants of less than twelve to eighteen months have none at all.

But the whole issue is not really as clear as we commonly assume. Other people's introspective testimony must pass through language, which in any case is essentially a behaviouristic vehicle. Even our own introspections, as soon as we start classifying and formulating them, owe to the same behaviouristic vehicle a degree of debt which would repay much closer scrutiny[1]. Furthermore, if we are to raise any philosophic objection to the postulates

[1] I have attempted this in the unpublished fuller study referred to earlier.

implicit in behaviouristic evidence, we must begin farther back with the very assumption that those ostensible physical objects, children, do exist independently of us and so are capable of having a psychic history of their own. To tangle up the issues still more, we have also to bear in mind all our contemporary discoveries of what a very fragmentary and imperfect picture even of our own experience our everyday unaided introspections tend to give us. Psycho-analysis has shown, first of all, what strong psychic obstacles there are to our getting access to large tracts of our own story, but secondly it has found the way to secure access to them, and so has provided us with an immensely enlarged and deepened picture of our psychic life and experience, by the side of which our ordinary one is obviously only a narrow and tendentious selection of fragments. And even without the specific technique of psycho-analysis there is ample material, of which it has pointed out the significance, in literature, anthropology, etc., in support of the same thesis.

(2) We cannot stop here to develop this discussion as it merits. We can only say, in general terms, that there is no difficulty in establishing such a relation between so-called behaviouristic evidence and our own experiences and states that in following the latter back towards the beginnings of our history, we can with full confidence lean more and more on the witness of the former, as fast as our direct testimony starts giving out. And our grounds for confidence have precisely the same force when applied first to the full " introspective " testimony, secondly to the diminishing verbal evidence as we go back to the first few years, and finally to the purely behaviouristic data of the beginnings of the history of other people. It is true that for these purposes we must postulate their existence, but this the whole tenor of our experience, as we have already seen, obliges us to do anyhow. Furthermore, if we prefer, we can quite as well tell the *entire* story in solipsistic terms ; we can treat it as wholly a reconstruction of our (my) own early experience-history, based on tracing backward everything we find in our developed psychic life and everything we can remember of its earlier stages and then merely completing the beginnings of the picture from what we can establish from all its later course.

The behaviouristic evidence about our early psychic history is of course both positive and negative, as well as buttressed by a great deal of more general observational knowledge. Everything we can note suggests and confirms, first, that from virtually the outset of our story a wide gamut of affective-conative experience is present, and secondly, that most of the modes and contents of what we should later call our cognitive experience remain for some time absent. We can mark the successive major events of visual exploration, auditory-visual co-ordination, hand-eye co-ordination, combined manual-visual exploration, learning to sit, to stand, to walk, and to talk ; and we can concurrently fill in and widen the picture of what the child becomes familiar with, from his narrowest immediate environment to a larger and larger circumambient world. What we have to do is merely to translate all this into experiential terms, with due care not to assume present in earlier phases anything that we can *watch being first introduced*, or barely and gradually emerging, at later stages. By the time we have completed our eliminating work, we are left with the postulate of an unintegrated, unclassified, purely qualitative early flow of experiences mainly affective-conative (distresses, cravings, reliefs, satisfactions), but showing also brief phases of a different kind. These go on without any strong nisus either way, but just sufficiently hold the child to make him prolong or continue them as far as he can and to let him discover increasingly that, unlike most of his more positive feeling states, they *can*, if he wishes, be carried on for longer and longer whiles.

(3) From something like that beginning, we can then observe all the rest following from the character of the child's successive experiences themselves, plus every new extension which we can see developing. It is important indeed to emphasise again that according to everything we know, experience has from the start the fundamental character of a *field* (or continuum), and not, as the early associationists tended (quite arbitrarily) to assume, of a punctate succession. And " field " does not mean here merely " spatial field," though this obviously comes into it (as an experienced character) almost at the outset. Even more fundamentally, the " field " as experienced forms part of a complex state, in which various qualitatively different elements are *co-experienced*, and co-experienced not only individually, but as at least two compresent but distinguishable (progressively self-distinguishing) *series*. There is on the one hand a succession of affective-conative states, themselves complex and overlapping ; there is, on the other hand, very often *concurrently with them*, a sequence of experiences of the kind we call perceptual (with their own focus-field structure). If the affective-conative state is intense, it thrusts everything else out ; if it is mild in degree, and a lively

perceptual experience occurs, this in turn may wholly absorb the child. But he may quite easily be conscious at the same time of both kinds. In effect, they increasingly come to distinguish themselves from one another both by their different quality and by their experienced separate development. (The difference in quality allows this separate development to manifest and to impress itself.) A particularly common and significant situation is that of one of the series remaining in a standstill or merely persevering phase, whilst in the other an active course of events is taking place. If it gets too active, the first, as we have said, fades out ; but we are all familiar with every degree of combination of both.

We can easily verify this from our current experience ; but the point here is that there is absolutely no reason, other than a parcel of gratuitous and arbitrary assumptions, for postulating anything different at the beginning of our experiential history. Vague misconceived early metaphors such as that of the *tabula rasa*, and crude notions about the " impact " of separate " stimuli " upon our " sense-organs," have led to a fantastic picture of our psychic life as a sequence of distinct sensations, or sense-impressions, registering themselves somehow, leaving copies, images or ideas of themselves, and then by repetition and habit getting associated with one another. This bears no likeness at all to what we find if we actually examine any of our experience, and is the substitution of wholly unsupported philosophic theory for the plain testimony of the facts. Thus it should be quite unnecessary to *disprove* that sort of view before we claim acceptance for that offered here ; on the contrary, the latter is what all our evidence demands and those who take the former (or any more sophisticated variant) should be challenged to state what grounds they think they have for it. And not only our own continual introspective findings, but all observation of the behaviour and expressions even of a baby only a few weeks old provide the amplest material for the same conclusion. There is endless evidence to show that he is constantly experiencing at one and the same time a complex tissue of feelings and desires, and (if these are not too strong) an equally complex but ordered pattern of perceptual experience, chiefly in the shape of focal attention to something he is seeing—within its own field—and more or less sustained following of it.

(4) To this picture of the so-called " stream of consciousness " in which two very different strains soon distinguish themselves both by their diverse quality and by their varying tempo, we

have to add, again within the first few weeks, at least one more experience-element, which thereafter renders the very notion of a " stream of consciousness " (or even of " experience " in its common, merely passive connotation) quite inadequate. This is once more the factor of activity, which expresses itself not only in movements of the body or limbs (not at first very significant psychically), but above all in those movements of the eyes which connote visual attention and become the first key to the whole development of the perceptual component in our experience. Our emphasis here is of course on the eye-movements merely as a cue, but primarily on the experienced psychic activity of visual attention. This rapidly becomes a major factor in the psychic life of the child, both in its own right and through the realms of further perceptual experience it is found to lead to. We need only touch again on the familiar psychological story of all the child's activities of exploratory visual attention and the ways in which these develop, sustain and organise his visual-perceptual field (or world) ; the concurrent growth of tactile attention and exploration, and the fundamental step by which the two fields are linked up and both brought under the one guiding visual control ; and the expansion of the visual-tactile field (into which auditory experiences have also been progressively integrated) through growing powers of movement and operative action, co-ordinated in turn with the developing sense of the child's own body, till the ensemble consolidates into a spatial arena all around him, of which he himself forms a part, and in which he lives and moves and has his being.[1]

(5) This is all common psychological ground, but philosophers concerned with the question of our warrant, if any, for believing in an external world are naturally not prepared to pay over-much attention to the ordinary way of telling the story which takes that world for granted and continually weaves it into the pattern of the child's development. On our own view that is in the last resort justified : the child's development is in fact a process of incessant interaction between himself as a psycho-physical existent and the physical world (including other psycho-physical existents like himself) around him. But unless we take great care about the way in which we bring the physical world in, we shall find that we have left a large and crucial part of the *psychological*

[1] It is not possible to consider here the special case of the congenitally blind child ; but it seems clear in principle that through the guidance of his psychic growth by seeing adults, he secures vicariously most of the benefit of their own visually controlled organisation of their experience.

story out ; that is in truth what usually happens and is the reason why the philosophers are entitled to regard the customary psychological text-book treatment of cognitive development as something extraneous and virtually irrelevant to their theme. What is essential even for the complete psychological story—and then manifestly makes it an indispensable prelude to the philosopher's theme—is to consider how far we can show *in terms of the child's own experience* (as pure experience) *how* he learns to regard himself as a psycho-physical entity, in process of incessant interaction with the physical world around him. And here we must take nothing for granted : not even the existence for him of the notion of the physical world, or of himself as a physical entity, or of any interaction between them. Our minimal problem, before we embarked on any assumption or theory, would be to try at least to establish the first time and mode of appearance in the child's thought of the above notions. In theory we might find ourselves compelled *in the end* to postulate their presence in some sense from the start. Or as we followed them back, we might come to a point where they seemed to make their début on our stage more or less fully fledged, without our being able to take their history back any further. Or we might find them ripening slowly during childhood, but by some mysterious inner process which we could only note but not understand. Or else—as we have discussed earlier—we might be able to demonstrate that they were a mere social heritage, a piece of gratuitous primitive metaphysical theorising which the child takes over unthinkingly from his human environment. Any of these alternative hypotheses *might* be true, but none must be taken for granted. In fact we shall find that none is needed or justified, because we can clearly exhibit the ways in which these notions, and the beliefs centred in them, are progressively pieced together by the child from the materials of his own experience and by the normal processes of that experience.

As we have already insisted, we are only assuming, at the beginning of the story, the child as experient (if one likes, ourselves as experients, or in the last resort myself as experient), passing through a range of diverse experienced states. At the end we have our (or my) world-picture, complete with physical world, human psycho-physical objects and these objects starting their psychic history with nothing but their own kaleidoscopic states, but ending up with that world-picture. Between that beginning and that end we shall find that we can demonstrate a complete sequence of processes and stages which lead from the one to the other, a sequence which we can express at each stage in terms for which previous ones have already prepared the ground and which thus they have already justified.[1]

That then is our subject-matter here. We can indeed claim that we are using our knowledge of the successive behaviouristic phases of early development only as a set of cues ; in particular, these cues call our attention, together with the data of our own memory and of the introspective testimony of others, to what we must *not* assume prior to each new phase. We must not assume, prior to the experiences of the mastery and exploitation of speech, all the expansions and articulations of our retained experiences which we can see evolving under the guidance and with the help of speech ; we must not assume prior to the experiences of the mastery of locomotion all the enlargements and articulations of experience which we can see being first contributed by this ; and so back to the experiences of the mastery of eye-hand co-ordination, etc., etc.

Our reconstruction of the growth and differentiation of our experience is thus in no way dependent on any extraneous assumptions. It is a reconstruction essentially from within, starting, as we have said, from a minimum of bare experiencing of our own states, and building up from distinctions and relations themselves progressively experienced, and the sheer cumulative extensions of our experience, all the structure which eventually we find. And if on account of the use we make, or appear to make, of behaviouristic or physical evidence, there should seem to be any doubt about the self-contained integrity of our experiential picture, the cross-sectional survey with which we began is intended to serve as a touchstone for this. It brings out that any and all of the distinctions or relations which our genetic account introduces can be uncovered or verified as experienced facts within almost any segment of our adult experience ; which still bears all its structural history, its tests and its sanctions, written within itself.

II.—THE CHIEF TYPES AND PHASES OF EARLY EXPERIENCE WHICH GO TO BUILD UP OUR WORLD-PICTURE

(6) Proceeding now with our thumbnail genetic sketch, we may pick out the following types and phases of our early experience

---

[1] A special tribute of acknowledgment is due here to the first chapter of the *Genetic Logic* of J. M. Baldwin, with its masterly presentation of a similar theme ; but nevertheless I have preferred to keep to my slightly different approach (which had been formulated before I became acquainted with the *Genetic Logic* twenty years ago) because it emphasises aspects of the story which even Baldwin's treatment does not, in my view, set in sufficient relief.

as without doubt the chief elements in the building up of our characteristic world-picture :

(1) *The first emergence of attentional objects in an attentional field :*

This is most readily and fully realised in terms of visual experience, though there are closely analogous (and very soon convergent) processes of tactile experiencing.

But even without going beyond the visual domain, the child finds that

(*A*) by suitable attentional activity and variations of such activity he can (*a*) maintain (*b*) relinquish (*c*) recover (*d*) extend particular experience-contents.   Through the continuity and increasing fusion of these experiences, together with the accompanying but distinct coefficient of directed attentional activity, there emerges their reference to a continuing attentional source. That is, the child is not merely having a *further similar* experience, but just as he can continue, so he can momentarily abandon but immediately recover the *same* content :   the same because it carries the same attentional coefficient, and because it goes on behaving as the identical content recovered and not merely as *another* similar one.   (There are plenty also of these.)   The notions of relinquishment and recovery develop of course *pari passu* with that of a continuing source turned to and turned away from by attentional variation.   All this begins very rudimentarily and uncertainly, but is quickly fortified first of all by unlimited repetition and so *repeatableness*.   And further by the possibility always of *extending* and *developing* the experience-content by the continued play of attention round the same focus or source :   which thus becomes more and more strengthened and consolidated *as* a focus or source.

(*B*) The attentional object or focus (source of a complex of experience-contents) which is thus " there " to be turned to has in any case an experienced field :   this is the original character of perceptual and in particular visual happenings, even if to begin with it only means that the experienced content has a more vivid portion, and a co-aware but less vividly co-aware *setting*.   This field enters closely into the experiences of relinquishing and recovering the original content, and indeed develops new foci of vividness as the previous ones are relinquished. Both the original field and its successive variations, including the new foci brought out, thus share in the status acquired by the original focus ;   they also are " there " in the same way, to be attended to and for attention to move in. In effect the further foci are relinquished and recovered turn by turn with the original ones, as the converse aspect of the same process. And through all this the status of all three participants in the process : the original focus, the alternative ones and the conjoining field, is further reinforced and extended.

(7), (11) *The development of attentional objects in the attentional field into " real " objects in a " real " (spatial) field :*

(*A*) The " thereness " of visual foci at various points (attentional directions) in a containing visual field is once more confirmed and strikingly expanded by a set of experiences which provides the inverse of all those linked with the child's own free attentional mobility. Sometimes when his attention is fixed upon a particular focus in a way which should maintain this, what happens is that on the contrary it starts fading away from him, just as if his own attention were moving away from it. But in fact in most of these cases he does not let this happen ; he struggles to retain the focal experience-content and finds he can do so by letting his attention *follow* it, i.e. move through the visual field with it. That becomes a first emerging coefficient of more than mere " thereness " ; of something like independent reality of those experience-foci or sources. They are no longer mere " objects " of and for attention; the child has now a distinctive experience as of foci or objects which move independently of attention, which pursue their own course and make attention follow this.

Again, the situation proves a common and oft-repeated one. As the experience recurs, it inevitably confers more and more of its own kind of reality also on the *field* in which it occurs. Attentional objects become, at least in a first degree, real objects, and the attentional field a real or spatial field. That realisation is carried further and fortified by the child's growing familiarity with (*a*) this continuing spatial field or setting in which his more specific experiences shift and change (*b*) the diverse foci or sources or objects in it (*c*) their habitual perceptual relations to one another within the field (*d*) the changes in those relations which go with the movements of particular objects, and (*e*) the experience of recovering or re-discovering familiar objects in different parts of the field from those they occupied before, i.e. as having moved (or, as he appreciates later, having been removed) from one relative position to another, even though he did not attend to or perceive their movement.

(8), (*B*) Concurrently with all this, various major new dimensions of " reality " build up round the same foci :

(*a*) Tactile perceptual experience, above all derived from manual activity, has established its own attentional objects— equally maintainable, recoverable, and capable of further development. These have from the start a specially powerful quality of their own, which subsequently enters deeply into our sense of " reality " ; they carry with them the experience of resistance, both as hardness and as counter-pressure (frequently to the point of immobility). But they likewise often provide a further dimension to the notion of mobility ; they do not indeed move away from the child's attention, but they lend themselves to the experience of activities of his own, by which he moves them.

These findings, however, remain relatively amorphous and unintegrated until, still within the first half of the child's first year, he learns to bring tactile and visual activity together, and the former in the main under the guidance of the latter. To each therefore accrues everything which the other is capable of contributing ; each gives support to the lessons of the other, whilst at the same time expanding and enriching them. The same experience-focus, or source, or now more than ever " object," can be seen, touched, handled, held, watched moving, moved by the child himself and watched as he moves it ; its reality now combines all these experienced attributes or dimensions.

(*b*) Auditory perceptual experience has even earlier proved largely capable of co-ordination with visual and so able to make its own contribution to the reality-content and reality-character of objects. The same applies, in lesser measure, to olfactory experiences and, with modifications, to those of temperature. The contribution of taste is of rather a different order, and comes under our next sub-heading below.

(*c*) The child's experiences of (i) his own bodily movements (ii) being moved, raised, lifted, carried (iii) the beginnings and developments of independent locomotion, combine with one another and with his attentional activities, first of all to enlarge and diversify his attentional field and its perceptual foci. And presently to take a stage further, both in content and in force, his sense of the all-round " thereness " of the field and of the specific " thereness " of particular foci at particular points within it. This process is of course immensely multiplied and fortified as independent locomotion is mastered and exploited ; in particular the pattern of seeing an object, moving towards it, touching and handling it, lifting and moving and removing it, is repeated scores of times each day in the most varied contexts. Objects become the more firmly objects, " there " and " real," with every day of successful manifold re-enactment of the pattern.

(*d*) The tale is carried further and endlessly reinforced as tactile and manual exploratory experience grows into more and more different forms of operative. Some of these are there very early and virtually inseparable from the most rudimentary tactile activities : squeezing, lifting and letting drop, waving, taking to the mouth and chewing, etc., etc. But it is only in the second half of the first year that they begin to get co-ordinated and directed and differentiated into a number of distinct, coherent behaviour-courses. Once this process is fully set going, however, it expands rapidly and almost without limit : activities upon objects, with objects, and with objects upon other objects become even more variegated than the objects themselves. And by the same token they prove capable of the fullest integration with the schemas of attentional, locomotive and visual-tactile perceptual experience to which we have already referred. Thus the " reality " of objects takes over in continuous and cumulative progression all the further ranges of meaning latent in their capacity for suffering changes from us and one another, and of effecting changes in one another—changes that vary from slight modifications to being broken up into their component elements on the one hand or being combined with others to the very loss of their identity. To be " real " now is to have real elements and to belong to an order of which the members are constantly liable to undergo real vicis-situdes and are constantly being used to bring about vicissitudes in one another.

(9), (III) *The integration into the given spatial field and among the acknowledged objects there of the special object which the child comes to think of as his own body.*

(*A*) On the one hand a large proportion of his experiences go to assimilate this object to all the others. First of all toes and feet and hands are continuing perceptual foci like the rest ; they too can be attended to visually and tactually, can be maintained, relinquished, recovered, and more fully explored ; they can be watched moving and moved towards ; and they are " there " in the same spatial field and the same way as toys, utensils, etc., etc. Secondly, the child learns in various ways to expand these more obvious foci to include more and more of his whole body, much of the surface of which he can take in visually and most of the rest tactually, whilst the sight of other complete human bodies and of reflections, etc., of his own familiarises him with the notion of this as a single object in its own right.

(*B*) On the other hand, a still greater proportion of the child's experiences converge to give this object a unique status in his world : it always stays an object and a body, but it also has a place and a meaning apart from everything else as *his* body. This special meaning is probably implicit from the start in a general organic awareness or sentience of his bodily life ; but at the beginning the full *perceptual* counterpart is lacking. The linking and fusing experiences between the child's progressive perceptual awareness and his organic sentience of his bodily life consist in the whole range of (*a*) all his physical pleasures and pains, often directly connected with perceived happenings in or to perceived parts of his body (*b*) his muscular and kinaesthetic experiences, which join up with all his perceptions of his hands and arms and feet, and eventually his whole body, moving and acting (*c*) his experiences of needs and cravings of which many are directly referred to particular bodily regions, and his experiences of satisfactions of these cravings which are again directly bound up with the same portions of his body (*d*) his gradual discovery that his perceptual experiences themselves, besides being linked up with a host of different foci or sources " there " away from and independent of his own states, have likewise all, without exception, another and distinctive linkage with certain perceived parts of his own body.

Even this is not the whole of an extremely complicated story which has never, I believe, been fully worked out ; but at any rate it exhibits some of the main experiential factors which amalgamate eventually to produce (i) our clear awareness of our body as a perceptual object, and finally a " real " object, like any other and among all others (ii) our clear awareness of these others as outside our body, at varying distances and directions from it (measured in the first place by movements of the trunk, the hands and our whole body towards them) (iii) our clear awareness of all these objects, including our own body and its various organs, as perceived through the suitable application of particular organs of that very body (eyes, hands, etc.) (iv) our clear awareness of our bodies as the seat and organ of all our feelings and desires and in the end also of all our experiences, thoughts, beliefs, memories, etc., and in fact of our whole psychic life (v) our equivocal shifting sense of our body sometimes as something external to our psychic self (" *my* body ") and at best only its instrument or vehicle, sometimes as the source and sole underlying reality of our psychic life, but mostly vaguely and fluctuatingly as something in between.

Our concern here is merely to describe, not finally to assess or to justify. There are true philosophic problems and mysteries arising out of the equivocal status of our bodies in our scheme of things ; we have already glanced at some of these and will do so again in our last chapter. But the psychological facts are clear, down to those of our equivocal attitude. And what is chiefly relevant for us here is what is clearest of all. Our experiences force us from the beginning and cumulatively throughout their course to acknowledge their perceptual contents as derived from foci or sources which are " there " independently of our own state but which, if by attention we subject ourselves to them, disclose themselves to us through those perceptual contents. However, this " thereness " becomes more and more interpreted, as our experience expands and develops, in terms not only of independence of our own momentary state, but also of spatial outsideness to and independence from our body as itself an object in space. This interpretation is made inevitable and continually re-supported by a myriad of findings of all the different kinds we have already described and have yet to enumerate. Nevertheless it can evoke queries and difficulties which we can only keep in their due place if we hold clearly in mind that the acknowledgment of the *psychological* independent " thereness " of our perceptual foci or objects is forced on us by irresistible experience prior to, and by a host of further experiences additional to, those which give rise to the picture of objects in space outside our own body as a spatial object. The latter picture is in the last resort derived from and sustained by the former experiences, not vice versa. And in the main, of course, it corroborates and reinforces them.

(10), (IV) *The development of the order of " real " occurrences or events concomitantly with the order of " real " objects, within a single objective world.*

(*A*) The original orders of experiences of the " perceptual " type, with their focus-field character, carry with them, under the auspices of the same coefficient of attentional activity, a component of experiences of *changes within* the perceptual focus or field. In contrast to the cases where part of the perceptual content changes as the attentional direction is *shifted*, there are various others where a change (also partial) occurs whilst the attentional direction remains *fixed*. But the shared features and large overlap of the two types of experience, side by side with their element of marked contrast, ensure their remaining linked together and undergoing a common, mutually supporting evolution, so that the child's developing picture of the objective world is always one of events which are really happening " there," as well as of objects which really exist (and persist) " there." This combination is the easier, since so large a proportion of the events the child watches are specifically happenings to or between objects, or enacted by objects.

(*B*) However, the growing acknowledgment of " real " happenings carries the child further, in several directions, into his objective world.

(i) He has to build up a clearer and clearer differentiation between the changes in his perceptual field which go with the movement of his attention, and those which occur while his attention is fixed : the former segregate out as happenings to him, changes in his perception, as contrasted with the latter which segregate out *pari passu* as happenings " there," perceptions of changes. This is not an easy distinction, since the latter are at the same time *also* changes in perception, or happenings to the child : the real difference is between perceptual happenings which have a dual status and those which have only a single one,[1] rather than between two wholly unlike types occurring in complete independence of one another, each in its own separate domain. Furthermore, the easiest cues to the distinction, the contrasted coefficients of moving and fixed attention, become blurred to some extent by the great class of cases of objects in motion which are changes or happenings in the " real " sense, but which are most characteristically taken in by means of moving attention, i.e. attention which follows the movement of the objects (as we have already seen). Finally, the child's habitual state comes more and more to be one of a continually fluctuating mixture of fixed and moving attention, with a corresponding medley of " mere " changes in perception and perceptions of real changes.

In spite of all these obstacles, however, the distinction is successfully carried through. This is the best measure of the amount of clear and effective support which it receives from the main

---

[1] In terms of *psychic happenings generally*, the difference is, strictly speaking, between those with a triple and those with a dual status, since the whole of our perceptual experience is distinguished by a dual one from all the rest of our " merely " subjective states. The latter are solely our experience whilst the former comes to stand out, as we have noted, as at the same time also experience that registers the existence and character of a world (*a*) of objects, *and* (*b*) of objective events.

character and course of our experiences themselves. Indeed, the contrasted coefficients of moving and fixed attention do not really fail the child even in the apparently ambiguous case of moving objects : we saw that he apprehends these through the *conjoint* experiences of stationary attention which loses its object (change in the perceptual content) and attention which retains this by moving indeed, but doing so under the control of the object. That is, by *following* it, and not shifting freely to and fro as in the typical exploratory mode (yielding " mere " changing perception). In the end, therefore, the child can combine the fixed and the mobile forms in all degrees and proportions, whilst yet clearly segregating those elements in the changing play of his experience which are only extensions or variations of his perception of unchanged things, both from such others as are perceptions of real changes in them and from those which are perceptions of real movements of *otherwise* unchanged things. His ability to discriminate between these different orders of experience is not indeed perfect on every occasion and in each detail ; but if occasionally he goes astray, he is soon pulled up and can usually learn to correct himself. Why ? Because in fact these different orders are there and confirm and consolidate our fundamental distinction between them in a way which turns every local error (through its correction) into further witness to its basic truth.

(ii) The distinction is in effect carried very much further for the child as there develops round each of the two main types of experience, i.e. perceived " *real* " happenings (including movements) and " *mere* " happenings-to-him (including his perceptions of real happenings) a separate and independent context of representations and beliefs. Perceived " real " happenings fall into recognised classes which he identifies by suitable portions of them ; but since they are temporal entities, he may identify one of a particular kind at a moment when a large part of it has happened already. Thus his perceptions of events carry with them a past context which belongs to *them*, not to the child. Or, taking the same process a stage further, he may perceive a state of affairs which he recognises as that usually left at the end of some familiar type of event or chain of events ; so that the whole of the latter helps to establish and fill out a past which is not the child's. And all these different pieces of a past which was " there," though not perceived at all, overlap and amalgamate eventually for him into a comprehensive objective past of events ; whilst this in turn coalesces with the past carried by the *continuance* of objects, into a single ensemble of past changes and persistences which finally becomes the inclusive fabric of (external or objective) History.

On the other hand " mere " happenings-to-him of the perceptual type join up, by endless cross-connections and overlaps, with all sorts of other " mere " happenings-to-him. This takes place all the time both as he goes along and also to an increasing extent by revival or recall, at first only of what virtually belongs to the still-lingering present, but gradually also of the less and less near past. Over against his developing picture of " real " happenings and their past and history, the child forms the context of happenings to himself, *his* past and history, initially in terms of his own retrospective memory, but ultimately as the sum-total of his story, whether remembered or not.

Of course what befalls himself is as real in its own right as what is occurring " there " in the objective world ; the child recognises this as he proceeds to take in the cross-relationships between the past of the world around him and his own, and to see the latter in its entirety as a specific course of events itself objectively happening within the larger context of the former. Yet this very insight merely acknowledges again that it is the order of objective occurrences independent of ourselves which remains the dominant fact, whilst what gives importance to the personal events which we call our successive perceptions is precisely their firmer and firmer status as information about the existences and occurrences in that objective world.

(iii) All these developments in turn fit into the actual patterns of our successive new perceptual experience and are fully borne out by this. And in virtue of that fact they open up more lines of advance for its further progressive organisation. In particular within the growing context of past happenings and the past history of this and that section of our world the child picks out recurring coherent themes which hold the fabric together and support and reinforce the reality of one another, and by the same token that of the context as a whole. This is of course the network of what we call causality, which will concern us more closely in our next chapter.

(11), (v)   *The building up of the full normal picture of our objective, spatio-temporal world with its diversity of occupants and occurrences and their total geography and history.*

The foregoing processes, by which the child shapes out of his experiences the pattern of the world which he is experiencing and *in* which he is experiencing, all go on concurrently and sustain and promote one another all the time. But they are far from the complete story yet and in fact they lead at an early stage to further differentiations which introduce powerful new dimensions of confirmation, whilst in addition they immensely expand and multiply the whole previous picture.

(*A*) Almost as fast as the child develops the sense of his recurrent and recoverable foci of perceptual experience as " real " objects in their own right, he becomes aware not only of his frequent refinding of the same ones, but also of the existence of numbers of more or less similar and more or less different ones. He gradually forms schemes of varying classes and sub-classes : rattles and other toys, cups and other crockery, socks and other clothing, and furniture and animals and humans. Many of the groups are further subdivided and a host of new ones are added as the child's range increases ; some in particular, such as that of animals and later of plants, prove capable of almost endless extension and refinement. On the other hand the human group consists primarily, in the earlier years, of a limited number of individuals cast for an outstanding role of their own, of which more later.

What applies to objects is found to be also true, even though not in the same measure, of events. Here too there are classes and sub-classes of similar occurrences (though in the nature of the case no recoveries of the same individual one : that of course is part of the main original experienced distinction in virtue of which the child shapes the separate categories of objects and events). The similarities again are of various degrees and contrast with varying degrees of difference.

In this more and more continuous surrounding world of objective entities and happenings with which he becomes increasingly familiar, and which he progressively sorts out and classifies and maps, the child gradually learns to recognise all kinds of further members and aspects. Besides discrete objects, he becomes acquainted with many other forms of substances, liquids, plastic materials, and eventually air and gases. In connection with all of these, he comes to note a variety of distinguishable recurring qualities, properties, states, parts, groupings and collections, situations, locations, etc. Besides more or less discrete events, he learns to acknowledge other forms of temporal happening, such as processes, occasions, cycles like day and night and the seasons, conjunctions and coincidences, etc. Linking up both objects and events, he becomes aware of endless different modes of relation and connection. All these and a vast number of other successive findings and learnings are seen to form recognisable classes, subclasses and wider classes, arrangeable in scales of resemblance and difference, and capable of being ordered in regular and more and more comprehensive hierarchies. The objectivity of the objective world holds good throughout the child's growing experience and learning and yields to this a wider and wider and richer and richer panorama of knowledge of itself.

(*B*) As and when he begins to be familiar with different *classes* of objects, substances, events, situations, occasions, etc., there enters into ever fuller functioning the combined process of recognition and anticipation, on which we dwelt in Chapter III. This operates on every level of specificity and generality, from the child's response to a particular kind of animal to his all-pervasive assumption that he is in a world of real things, in all the senses of " real " which we have described. With recognition and anticipation, there comes on the one hand the possibility of pre-adjustment and, as widening schemes of representation are formed, the building up of more and more elaborate patterns of action and of planning based on the assumption that various such schemes (both local and larger) are correct ; but on the other hand, there comes also the possibility that to a greater or lesser extent, some of these schemes may be found wrong. We have already emphasised how this experience in turn provides a fundamental further dimension of " reality " for the world of " real " objects and occurrences, enforced directly through their perceptual manifestations. The latter become now the hard or real *facts* which test whether the child's recognitions and anticipations, beliefs and representations, are true or false ; the facts to which, if they are to be true, they must conform. These beliefs, however implicitly and absolutely he may have read their substance into the nature of things, are now relegated to the status of something merely pertaining to him : parts of his personal history, and nothing more. If they are not borne out by the perceptions which actually come to the child, they must be corrected or changed. Wherever necessary, new and true beliefs have to be formed. The limits of resemblance of different classes of things, events, etc., have to be learnt, and truly learnt. The characters and properties that go together and those that do not have to be learnt, and truly learnt. And ignorance, i.e. a gap or lack in our expectation-scheme, failure to provide for something " there " in a given situation, can be quite as disastrous as error : the child has to get to know not only what to expect of particular classes of objects, events, situations, etc., but also what classes of objects, events, situations, etc., to expect in every sort of context into which he is apt to be brought.

(*C*) This process, if it is followed out to any extent, involves further and further penetration both into the geographical and temporal distribution and into the nature and properties of things ; and eventually also into their history. The recognition that objects and events have a past of their own and form part of an endlessly receding history is not only borne out directly by the possibility of further explorations which in fact fill in more and more of that past and that history. The same recognition, and the ensuing fuller knowledge of the past, also proves the key to a truer and more complete picture of the behaviour and deploy-ment of things in the future, and so to the possibility both of more far-reaching and of more successful plans of action.

(12), (*D*) But these more advanced extensions of the child's field of knowledge and of vision and prevision do not come until he has made much progress with the exploitation of a much earlier piece of fundamental learning. Among the real objects he comes to recognise and acknowledge there are some which, as we have said, are outstanding in importance for him. These are obviously the human beings round him, and presently we shall be more specifically concerned with the pivotal figures among them. Here we wish rather to bring out certain features common to them all and of pregnant significance for all the further growth of the child's picture of his world.

(i) He finds, separately but convergently, that (*a*) they are extremely similar to him in many ways (*b*) he is extremely similar to them. (Sometimes he starts from one end, sometimes from the other ; and because he has not the advantage of directly seeing the logical implications of the relation of similarity, he has the excitement of making the discovery twice over, once from each side.)

The close resemblances prove to be twofold : other humans are bodily objects like himself, and he like them ; and they have experiences like his, whilst he has experiences like theirs. These two sets of findings greatly soften and indeed go far to remove the antithesis between himself and the objective world, both in its psychological and in its bodily aspect : there is now direct continuity between himself, as object and as subject, and all the rest of the world he comes to acknowledge and to learn to know.

There are objects like himself in the essential sense that they are also persons, who see and think and feel just as he does—who are in fact equally, as he gradually comes to see, subjects confronting a world which they can only get to learn about, but must learn about, from their own experiences and states. Yet they are also *objects* in all the same senses as any of those other perceptual foci which he discovers as continuing and " there," and as real features in a continuing and " there " and real world. And at the same time it turns out that there is a regular gradation of characters, behaviour and properties, from these objects so like the child himself (even as subject) down to all those inanimate things which initially seem to have nothing in common with him (and though he has to acknowledge their existence, appear to exist in a different way from himself, and indeed only in an inferior one). This then in turn places himself too as an object in the same series, existing like the rest in the same world ; and eventually he realises that that is just how he does present himself to other subjects like himself.

(ii) What is, however, far more important to him than the train of findings which leads more or less implicitly, and comparatively slowly, to the foregoing conclusions, is his early and immensely significant discovery that it is possible to share actual experiences or states with these other objects, which prove to have similar experiences and states to his own.

No doubt this is more than a discovery : we may well assume that there is something organic and innate in himself which expresses itself from the start in his relation with his mother and in all his interchanges with her—something which probably facilitates each further stage of his growing awareness of his communion with other human beings (that is, his responses to the manifestations of their psychic states and their responses to the manifestations of his). But whilst we do not have to deny or disparage this probability, we do not in any way need to lean on it. All the elements for a cumulative *experiential discovery* such as we have described are *there*, and would be sufficient. Moreover it is plain that the scope for direct communion on an innate basis is strictly limited and, as experience shows, such communion or assumed communion is quite prone to error. In the main the child's full realisation of the sharability of his experiences with those of other human objects depends for most of its concrete material on his thoroughly empirical acquisition of the communicating medium of language (itself, as we know, a tremendous discovery). And this applies with the greatest force to the types of experience with the sharability of which we are here specially concerned ; the experiences of perception, recollection, anticipation and representation.

(iii) There is much that is of great interest, which we cannot stop to work out here, about the actual process and stages by which the child is inducted into the assumption (far from self-evident) that other people's cognitive (perceptual and other) experiences are like his own. But in fact the assumption works and completely justifies itself. And the first key development which we should note is the child's discovery of the far-reaching *interchangeableness*, or mutual substitutability, of his perceptions, recollections, anticipations and representations with those of the humans round him. He can base *his* anticipations on *their* perceptions or their recollections, as well as their actual anticipations. And they can do the same thing in relation to him. There is, as it were, a common human currency or pool of experiences and information on which the child himself, and everyone else, can draw in substitution for his own, at any point where there is a gap, with the same overall validity (even if also with the same occasional fallibility).

(iv) Finally, there follows from the foregoing the great transforming consequence that the child can endlessly enlarge and multiply the scope of his own experience by drawing on all the pool of that of the people round him. He is not dependent *only* on what he can learn from the sequences, the conjunctions and combinations, the developing patterns, of his own experiential history ; he can take over ready-made almost anything he wants to know that has already been learnt by others, who so visibly moreover have far greater powers of every kind than he has himself. In the end he finds that there is thus open to him (in a civilisation such as ours) the greatest part of what has been learnt throughout its history by the whole race of men.

(13), (E) The crucial point of these progressive discoveries of the child, from our angle, is that they all rest on his acknowledgment of the independent existence of a world which is found to embrace many other objects like himself, that is, similar in every aspect, including the possession of an experience-life like his own. That acknowledgment is thus further corroborated and reinforced by the whole body of confirmations and successes and new extensions to which this one application of the principle leads. There are firstly, as we have seen, the direct uses of the communicated anticipations of others for successful anticipations of the child's own ; it is thus evident that these others have the same sort of picture of the same objective world—and are equally right in their belief in this. But beyond these specific and immediate bearings-out of the child's own picture which he takes for granted, we can watch the far more gradual and explicit processes by which he comes to grasp that his own picture can be expanded in range and enriched in content in every direction by deliberately drawing on all the wider knowledge about that same objective world possessed by his more advanced fellow-dwellers in it. In the same process he learns of course also that they were once as he is, and that he is on his way to becoming as they are. All this fits together again and everything supports and strengthens, even as it continually enlarges, his picture of the one shared objective world, there to be taken in and explored and learnt about by everyone. Thus even the very course of his own learning from experience, which is so fundamental for him, now takes its rightful place in the objective scheme of things as only a small instance of a vastly larger similar learning process carried on over an immense period of time by myriads of entities like himself within the same objective world. And by the same token the latter now becomes something of which our only interim measure is the sum-total of all that the race has come to know about it so far, but which still surpasses that sum-total to an unfathomable extent since the process of learning is still, in all directions, going on.

(*F*) It might appear that the foregoing exaggerates the degree of support of the child's reading of his own experience which he can legitimately draw from the communicated information of others, since after all most of the latter is for him mere hearsay, the correctness of which he has no means of verifying. Moreover, it may be said, and has been said, that his own interpretation is almost from the beginning heavily coloured by that hearsay and comes to consist more and more predominantly of this : from about his third year onward, he is being supplied all day long with communicated information and a communicated general scheme of things, and indeed it is only with the help of these that he is able to build up eventually the characteristic human (= social) world-picture he does.

We have already provided most of the material for answering any such objections, which are essentially based on not examining the facts. Even before the child can begin to turn for aid to communicated information, he has gone through an immense cumulative learning process in which the main underlying structure of his future world scheme has already taken shape. It is true that without any help from language and from all this brings, the scheme would remain something merely assumed and enacted and lived, rather than something thought and represented. But the crucial fact is that even when language has come on the scene and when (rather later) the process of social communication of the locally accepted world-picture has begun to operate in strength, all the direct learning processes are continuing their fundamental work. Moment by moment the child is carrying on the cycle of attending and perceiving, anticipating, moving and acting in the light of this, and again attending and perceiving. Moment by moment he is thus bringing into operation what he has already learnt about the import of his perceptual experience not only in the shape of both specific and general expectations, but also in that of more and more elaborate purposive action built on these. And moment by moment everything he is thus relying and acting upon is undergoing the new (and transcendent) test of the further primary perceptual experience which actually comes or happens to him. And this, as we have noted, continually verifies his system of anticipations in the main ; indeed, even whilst it frequently falsifies some local feature, it does so in a way which further confirms the system as a whole (that is, the fundamental belief in an objective world).

A large part of the information socially communicated to the child, above all in his earlier years, enters in fact, either immediately or sooner or later, into the same self-testing process. It leads to characteristic expectations and adjustments directed to his further experience, and becomes subject to the latter's verdict. It is in effect mostly again verified, else the child's current behaviour, and still more his further growth in powers of adjustment and purposive action, would break down. As his social education goes on, the proportion of information which is not subjected to any direct experiential test, at least in any immediate form, increases at an accelerating rate, but so of course does the child's built-up knowledge based on his own experiences, and equally (under suitable educational conditions) his power of judging, at least roughly, the degree of dependability of different kinds of communicated information. Indeed, as this is derived at different times from many different social sources, these serve, at least in some degree, as a *check on one another*, since the experience of the clash of a belief *previously* accepted with information, or alleged information, *now* offered acts as a challenge for further inquiry as to which is right. The final test is then usually, directly or indirectly, the verdict of primary perceptual experience. Moreover there is little that is socially believed (if it really *is* believed) which does not, in one form or another, enter eventually into our current representations or expectations in some field of current actual experience and thus become subject to the testing action of the latter.

It is true that this action can be avoided or evaded in various ways. The whole theme is a complex one, with far-reaching implications, which cannot be pursued here. It is important only to recognise that provided a sufficient proportion of our social beliefs are correct enough for ordinary practical purposes (i.e. provided that the specific anticipations based on these are in fact borne out), there is always room for quite a large admixture of undetected, or at any rate uncorrected error. In earlier cultures, indeed, particularly in the more primitive ones, the minimal true world-picture which must be formed for survival usually supports a great superstructure of part wishful, part fearful fantasy operating in ways that actually preclude any direct and decisive experiential tests. Nor is our own society quite free from a fringe of similar inherited pensioner beliefs. But by and large the greatest part of what the child learns socially in our own mainly scientific civilisation is in fact upheld by the same criteria as those by which his own fundamental belief in the objective world around him has been formed and tested and re-tested beyond any real possibility of doubt. Most of this information is, moreover, still being continually re-tested and re-confirmed all round the child, if not by himself ; and the vast enlargement of his own picture thus brought about, together with everything he successfully builds on it, provides him with the most effective further verification and reinforcement of his basic beliefs.

(14) We have now covered most of the essential ground and may very briefly glance back over our main course so far, before we add to the story a final chapter needed to introduce a certain correction of perspective—a correction which again supports, at the same time as it qualifies, our broad picture.

The child's individual passage from " mere " personal experience to the belief in a world of objects independent of experience can be exhibited schematically in the following progressive stages, each flowing continuously out of the one before and flowing continuously into the one after :

(i) experiencing of the " perceptual " type or quality

(ii) specific contents attended to and perceived

(iii) specific foci felt to be " there," attended to and perceived

(iv) specific foci " there " *to be* attended to and perceived

(v) specific foci or " objects " " there " before they were attended to and perceived, and " there " after they cease to be attended to and perceived

(vi) specific objects " there," whether they happen to be attended to and perceived, or not—and following their own course, acting upon others and acted upon by them, irrespective of us and our attentional, perceptual or other activities

(vii) objects " there " even if they are never perceived or are out of the reach of perception, as part of an objective world which extends in every direction (of space and time) far beyond our powers of perception.

Belief, over and above immediate experiencing, enters already between phases (i) and (ii) and then passes almost imperceptibly into (iii), in virtue above all of the child's attentional experiences, and his discovery of the recoverableness, and so of the continuing character, of the contents perceived. This belief, as expectation, is constantly confirmed and consolidated, and soon expands, through the various other experiences we have noted, into the successive further stages from (iii) to (vii). And whilst, as we have seen, it starts most readily from the easiest cases of " some (persisting) thing there " in the shape of objects, it quickly picks up also the closely affiliated other series of experiences of " some change there " or " some happening there," which becomes the order of objective events and fuses with that of objects in our one comprehensive common sense and scientific picture of our " real " world.

The significant thing about the whole progression is that each stage builds upon all those before, and as it is in turn verified by the further course of experience, it adds the most striking and powerful confirmation to all the main structure of beliefs formed before. Having found them true, the child carries them on another stage, in a way which is only *possible* because they are in fact true. And then the same thing happens again, and subsequently again, each time providing new proof that the course followed so far must have been right, since on each occasion it opens out still further in the same direction.

The "objects" which the child discovers to be "there" to be attended to and perceived *prove* to be also objects to be moved towards even when not perceived, objects to be acted upon, objects to be acted with, objects acting on his own body, objects acting on one another, objects with their own past and future, objects to be reckoned with in any picture of his own past and future, etc., etc. Each successive one of the further experiences described in these ways gives fully *congruent* additional substance and depth to the child's first reading of the conjunction of his attentional activities and his perceptual experience as attention to and perception of objects "there." He forms a wider and wider and more and more detailed picture of the object world, and in the measure in which he does so, he finds himself able to plan and carry out more and more elaborate series of movements and actions based upon that picture and linking up with different portions of it in ways which themselves depend on the whole picture being borne out. His plans succeed in effect, in so far as the picture does prove correct ; and this happens often enough to allow him continually to develop his plans of action still further and to superimpose new ones on the old. But at the same time it is constantly being demonstrated to him, by a certain proportion of actual errors and also by all-too-frequent experiences of not being able to foresee or plan beyond a certain point, that his picture represents only a fraction, and in part an imperfectly dependable fraction, of *what is there to be pictured*. And thus all these experiences confirm still more strongly the correctness of his fundamental belief that there is a world "there" which can be attended to and found out about— and which imperatively demands this fealty from him if he is to go about *any* of his ways in safety and with success.

We can say that by and large this is the end-result which, in our scientific dispensation, a growing proportion of the population reaches. But (as we have already noted) it is not, in any fully generalised form, attained in most pre-scientific communities, and it is not attained in that form without effort and qualification even in ours. To bring into our story the main reasons for this, we must now introduce the qualification referred to above.

(15) We have not so far directly considered either the mode or the stages of emergence of one most important order of relationships of our perceptual experience to other types ; an order which is in many ways the most distinctive and important of all. It is that of control of the comings and goings of most if not all

of our affective-conative experiences, both positive and negative. This character of our perceptual experience has of course entered either implicitly or explicitly into most of our previous description, especially of the later stages of the child's developing relation to his world. But there are features about its earlier phases which demand our particular attention.

One of the first and most compelling lessons learnt by him is that the satisfaction of his cravings and needs, the achievement of innumerable forms of pleasure, and his relief from endless pains and distresses are completely bound up with the presence or absence of specific sets of perceptual experiences. That is naturally a gradual discovery, but it goes on cumulatively the whole time, in terms both of continual repetitions of the same kind of case and of the incessant occurrence of new ones. Typical perceptual experiences usher in the gratification of his needs and to a greater or less extent accompany this ; and it constantly happens that at the same time as he loses them, his gratification is cut off and his affective state is suddenly transformed into its opposite. On the other side various typical perceptual experiences are encountered together with specific pains and discomforts, but as the former lapse, the latter disappear with them. And again, the child meets with new constellations of perceptions and finds that either they carry with them direct pleasure, or they quickly become linked with activities on his part which bring new satisfactions to him (toys, foods, sweets, etc.).

All this is reinforced and developed as the initial sets of happenings to the child crystallise into experiences of continuing foci and of objects. The perceptual world becomes more and more clearly a world of real and independent entities and occurrences, on the presence, absence and vicissitudes of which the child's own states of gratification and frustration, pleasure and pain, happiness and unhappiness, entirely depend. Their " reality " acquires the all-important further dimension of prepotent control over everything that matters most to him within his own feeling states. His whole will and strivings and his more and more elaborate purposive activities become trained upon a selection of heterogeneous objects, occurrences and situations in the objective world, of which he has to try somehow to secure the presence or realisation or regular recurrence, or alternatively to control the absence, if he is to be at ease or peace or contented within himself. Thus in acknowledging the existence of the objective world, he must at the same time learn to acknowledge his dependence upon different objects or components within it for his own most vital feelings and wishes and needs. And this is a dependence which, as we have already seen, means in fact that he must set out to learn more and more about that world—both the characteristics of the particular components that matter to him, and their relationships to their setting and to his own bodily situation and circumstances. For only so can he also go on to learn the right sequences of activities on his part (locomotive, operative and every sort of other behaviour) in order to bring himself, physically and psychically, into that relation to them which will yield him the feeling states he seeks.

Yet although this emerges in a thousand forms from the child's earliest days, and he cannot help drawing most of the right conclusions, the pattern comes to him with a certain heavy bias and with many confusing and misleading elements. These cannot indeed nullify the main tenor of his experience, but they can and do lead him *partly* astray, in some cases for a long time, and in others for good.

The heavy bias arises because, though he has ample opportunities of building up his sense of perceptual objects in terms of his cumulative experiences of a host of specimens of every sort about him, there is in fact one single, preferential, central one round which all that is *most important* in his early psychic life revolves. The child's most powerful and impressive first learning from his experience (which, as it happens, includes a great deal of mislearning) must inevitably be in terms of that first pivotal object, his mother. Here is his most significant first continuing, recoverable, recurring focus of perceptual experiences ; here is an " object " which moves out of his field and comes back into it, which can be followed as it moves, and watched as changes or happenings occur in it or in relation to it ; here is an object which acts on his body, and on which he acts with various parts of his body, etc., etc. And above all, here is a perceptual object with the presence and activities of which are bound up all his most vital affective states, cravings, distresses, reliefs and satisfactions.

Thus the child has the opportunity of building up, in all the ways we have described, his notion of and scheme of beliefs in this outstanding object, just as he does in the case of lesser ones. We may probably assume, indeed, that there is a deep initial bond with far-back organic roots which from the beginning gives the infant's experiences of his communion with his mother a *sui generis* quality—a quality that might well carry with it some sense of both separate and complemental *existence* ; an experience of striving towards, which projects or postulates something there to be striven towards. But we do not have to depend in any way on such an assumption ; the child, as we can easily see, has an overwhelming amount of experiential material which would in any case, within a very short time, lead up to the acknowledgment and full notion of the central object round which most of his experience becomes organised. And whatever initial quasi-organic sentience there may be, we can in fact judge from the behaviouristic and expressional evidence that it takes some little time before the infant has sorted out and stabilised, from among the general flux of his experiences, a sufficiently articulated sense of his mother as an entity in her own right, to be able to respond to her as such. It is only in the course of the second month that we get that first unmistakable sign of the recognition of the mother as a person, the beginnings of a welcoming smile. After that, all the child's experiences marshal themselves round this recognition and give it more and more substance and scope. Everything confirms and develops it. The comings and goings and activities of this dominant object in the child's world are found to control in one way or another, at least at the outset, practically everything that matters to him.

Yet whilst she is thus the pre-eminent power in his immediate universe, it is still true and very important for his unfolding world-picture that she appears as an " object " (for attentional and perceptual experience and every sort of object-directed activity) among others, and in many ways like any and all of them. There are no few such " object " foci which he notes and watches in the field in which she herself moves ; and there are a multitude to which she introduces him, in the course of tending him, feeding him and playing with him. Some of these are left with him and he has the opportunity of exploring them and acting on them and with them in the characteristic ways that build up his full notion of " objects " as such.

Moreover, though it is true that the mother appears as a different sort of being from these others in even more ways than she resembles them, it is also true that she does not long retain her unique character and status. We have already noted the significant existence of a series of more or less intermediate objects, representing a broadly continuous scale of degrees of resemblance and difference, down to the inert things which at first seem to offer the maximum contrast to that great living power. Close to her, there are all the other personal objects, some of which progressively loom larger but which keep multiplying and diverging in their degree of likeness : first father, brothers, sisters, other relatives, nurses, etc., then gradually the rest of the human world. Not so far away from this world of human objects there is that of the animals, which, however, is found to cover a vast range that eventually moves far away from the human domain and in some respects may seem to come within hailing distance of the realm of non-living objects round the child. These in turn offer their own apparent bridges and passages : lifelike toys, machines that seem to have their own powers of movement, objects with mysterious properties like magnets, etc., etc.

So that before very long, say by about the child's fifth year, he has a comprehensive picture of an objective world full of all manners of creatures and things, with the most varied characters and properties, from humans, human-like animals and quite different animals to plants and engines and inert objects. But all of them taken in through perception and learnt about by more perception and all having the characteristics of being objects, i.e. objective independent existences in their own right with their own place and past history and relationships and future course.

(16) However, the fact that his first central experience of the most important object in his world and his subsequent experience of the next most important ones is throughout of the same personal type leaves its strong impress on his developing picture of the world. On the one hand the comings, goings and activities of these pre-eminent entities seem to be infinitely varied, incalculable and governed only by themselves. Other objects are at their beck and call, and mostly passive and inert until acted upon or acted with by these personal powers. On the other hand the latter can to some extent be influenced, in the direction wanted by the infant, by the bare expression of his needs and wishes (by cries and even by mere looks), in ways which are completely ineffectual with most other objects, especially all inert ones. Sometimes indeed the wishes themselves seem to be enough ; they are no sooner felt than the mother is already acting to satisfy them.

Since the child can only read his world in terms of his experience of it, he starts with a strong sense of overriding personal beings for which the rest of the scheme of things provides the means and instruments. This is complicated but not contradicted if a little later on he begins to interpret inert things themselves more or less in his own likeness, as being somehow alive and having some inner personal being of their own ; these inert things still remain dependent upon the greater human powers and subject to their will.—Any such automatic reading of the world is indeed gradually counteracted, or at least restricted and qualified, by further experience showing the limited writ of the personal beings round the child. There are many objects and occurrences which they cannot control and to which he finds them as subject as he himself is. Even those which they can control sometimes get manifestly out of hand, or at some point resist, or he observes that even his mother or father or other surrounding human powers can only get the better of them by laboriously *learning* to do so.

On the other hand, however, the child has many further encounters which seem to confirm and extend his sense of personal powers imposing their own designs on things, bending them to their purposes, intervening in them and directing them. And there are also various patterns of *imaginings* arising from many powerful impulses and desires and fears, which are so vivid and strong that they irresistibly turn themselves into actual beliefs in the existence and pervasive presence of *unseen* personal beings, directly derived from or very much like the human ones on which all the child's early life turns. Whilst in addition of course he comes more and more under the influence of prevailing social doctrines which very often give definite forms and further potent suggestive authority to just such beliefs.

Acted upon by the foregoing factors and other cognate ones (which cannot in this thumbnail sketch be elaborated) at the same time as by his main objective learning history, the child has little choice but to emerge with a more or less vague and confused total picture. This has been all too apparent in every culture prior to our own, but still applies to some extent even in ours. In that picture a more or less large domain of definite acknowledgment of everyday practical objects and occurrences with their own characters and properties and rules which in the main can be directly learnt and adapted to is surrounded by a great penumbra of human-like personal beings with overriding powers, which may intervene anywhere at times, but in any case have their own special haunts or realms in which we must ascertain their will and adapt to them. However, the history of our particular civilisation has shown most conclusively that this sort of picture is not the last word of what there is to be learnt from our human experience.

D*

It has become clearer and clearer that if the processes by which we build up the *non-personal* part of our world-picture are freed from all obstructing, arresting and deflecting influences, if we go on attending and exploring, observing, comparing and experimenting, and in every way consistently acting on the *assumption* of an enduring and thus learnable non-personal world order, we can in fact extend our non-personal picture indefinitely. And in so doing we can be assured of its continual further verification and confirmation, both by direct correspondence of primary perceptual experience (observation) with anticipation or belief, and by more and more powerful and successful controlling activities based on such beliefs.

We must note then that a full account of the history of our experience has to take cognisance not only of an immense amount of cumulative *true* learning, but also of a considerable element of plausible and tenacious and far-reaching *false* learning, which, however, we can and do gradually learn to correct. And the process of correction, very significantly and illuminatingly, proves to be in essence a re-affirmation and wider application of the original modes of cumulative learning based on the acknowledgment of an objective world and unremitting attentional-perceptual submission to it. As part of this process the prepotent personal powers round the child eventually become ordinary finite human beings like the subject himself (and he like them) among myriads of others, present, past and future ; whilst most of their magnified shadows and ghosts, left with less and less anchorage, place and power, progressively fade out. At the same time all human beings come to be seen as just members of one particular sub-class of the great and infinitely diversified class of living things. And this in turn is recognised as only one subdivision of the vastly greater class of physical objects (or systems) at large. Whether our fully sifted experience, embodying the cumulative outcome of all our secular learning processes, discloses any evidence for the presence after all of some ultimate personal power is a question beyond the scope of this psychological sketch ; but at any rate the strong predisposition towards such a view which most of us have carried with us from our childhood provides no valid reasons in its favour, but has on the contrary had to give further ground with every successful new advance in our knowledge based on an approach which completely disregards it.

(17) If now, in the light of our last few sections, we cast a final glance over the child's cognitive history as it actually unfolds,

without seeking to marshal the facts to bring out any particular thesis, however important, it is clear that our true start should be from the central cycle of his developing interchanges with his mother (that is, the cycle of experiences which we as observers describe in these terms, but from which the child has first to learn the distinctions and relations embodied in the very description). Round this cycle, and for a while as very much subordinated to it, we should have to group first his other important personal relationships and only secondly the further incidental undergoings and doings which enter into his slowly growing intervals of wakefulness and alertness. In trying to reconstruct the actual course and balance of his experiences, in order to pick out the threads of his cognitive growth, we should pay a duly weighted regard not only to the evidences of the movements and arrests of his attention, but also to his far more emphatic manifestations of feeling and all his bodily movements and activities (not omitting, with conventional Grundian blindness, his basic bodily functions, which the psycho-analysts have obliged us to view in their proper large place in the infant's psychic life). Yet out of all the initial confusion and anarchy of his experiences and feelings we should still see gradually emerging the progressive expressions of his increasing powers and achievements of co-ordination, organisation and integration. And even from the central cycle of experiences alone we could show crystallising out, feature by feature and relation by relation, the notion of an object and of other objects ; the notions of movements and other happenings ; the notion of the dependences of feeling-states on the right objects and happenings ; the notion of all the continuing goings-on round the child, his own bodily undergoings and doings, the doings and undergoings of other objects like himself, and the doings and undergoings of objects unlike himself ; the notions of regular courses of events and of recurrent groupings of both objects and events in characteristic situations and occasions, etc., etc.

At the same time, however, we should also show how all the flanking cycles of experiences make their own supporting contributions ; and how these in fact become more and more distinctive and those cycles broader and broader, more and more separate and increasingly dominant, till the initially paramount one becomes in turn quite subordinate and its share in the child's picture of his world—at any rate in our (more or less) scientific civilisation—minor by comparison with that of all the rest of his experience. And we should be able to exhibit how by continuous

stages this wider experience leads to the discrimination and acknowledgment of a greater and greater diversity of objects, objective
entities and happenings, and their parts, aspects, states, relations
and groupings ; how, as we have already noted, objective substances come to range up to the apparent insubstantiality of air
and gases, and objective entities can be as unlike primary objects
(or even entities) as streets or farms or schools, valleys, waterfalls,
and presently geological strata or faults, sunspots, or the iono-
sphere ; how room has eventually to be found among objective
facts or factors for such actualities as the British constitution, the
religion of Ancient Egypt, the nineteenth century, surface tension,
blood groups, etc., etc. And finally throughout this whole evolution we should have to note the triple fact that (i) perception continually maintains and consolidates its paramountcy as the
sovereign means alike of extension and of test of our beliefs, but
(ii) what is immediately perceived becomes a smaller and smaller
nucleus in a constantly expanding context or system of beliefs
(consisting of assumed compresent context as well as assumed past
and inferred future), and (iii) the *occurrence* of perception becomes
more and more detached from the content perceived, more and
more extraneous, contingent and virtually irrelevant, because we
know from past learning that under the conditions of scientific
discipline and control of perception, the content perceived is
equally valid (is expressive of the objective scheme and nexus of
things) whether we chance to be attending to it or not. Of course
perception must occur, so that *we* may secure its content, and we
must see to it that it occurs as copiously, systematically and
searchingly as possible. But that is only so that *we* may attain
adequate and accurate knowledge, and this is knowledge precisely
because its content holds good whether we possess it or not. In
so far as it is genuinely established and tested, it is knowledge of
what objectively is and happens, or has been or has happened, or
will be or will happen, irrespective of whether or not we have
come to know of it.

(18) At the end of this sketch we are logically brought back to
the crucial point established in an earlier chapter : the most fundamental dividing line of all in our experience is not that between
the *total* " perceptual " portion of it (which of course at any particular time is mostly derived from our past) and the rest, but
between the whole of our history, including all past perception
and its outcomes and products, up to any given moment, and the
new perceptual experience which comes after that moment. Every-

thing with which we confront this new happening to us, our retained past perceptual experience and the information and beliefs we have gathered from this no less than any other element in our state, is now clearly and irremediably subjective ; my beliefs are *my* beliefs, as surely as my feelings are my feelings. And our new perceptual experience impinges on all this as something extraneous, uncontrollable and irresistible, which may or may not fit in. If it does not, then, as we have seen, it breaks through our prepared pattern, imposes itself and forces us to change our previous beliefs in whatever way may be necessary in order to accommodate it.

This new perceptual experience thus manifests directly the objective order which we have been seeking to know, and acts as a continuous series of running tests of whether the beliefs we have so far come to form, the supposed information or knowledge we have gathered up to the moment, are as adequate and accurate as we assume them to be. The test is constantly varied ; from instant to instant it catches our system of pre-existing beliefs at different points and in different ways. The actual *new* perceptual content at each moment is, as we have seen, only a minute fragment by comparison with the context of beliefs worked by the immediately preceding perception, into which it fits or fails to fit. The same applies to the further context of beliefs which in turn it stirs into action in preparation for and anticipation of the next fragment of actual perception. Yet each of these successive coloured or patterned fragments (like bits of a jigsaw puzzle : mostly visual, though with a certain amount of tactile, pressure, temperature, auditory and other sensory patternings interwoven) does most clearly and definitely match, or refuse to match, the relevant portion of our pre-existing belief or information scheme, and any five minutes' changing perceptual experience involves an uncountable number of distinct tests of different portions of that scheme.

We have noted that though there are frequent misfits, of varying degrees and kinds, and though these in the nature of the case loom very large when they actually happen, they are only an infinitesimal fraction, in our ordinary life, of all our incessant passages, smooth and unnoticed, from true fit to true fit. In other words, an immensely preponderant proportion of our current scheme of beliefs is a true reflection (in terms, of course, of our perceptual medium) of the objective order which impinges on us in the specific so-ness of each moment's new perceptual experience, and we have therefore in the main nothing to fear from each such new impingement, even though every new turn in it tries our scheme at a new point and in a new way.[1] We do, as we have insisted here, get our jars and shocks, which from time to time may be severe ; but by comparison with our total scheme of beliefs, even the severest ones usually prove to be (at least intellectually !) only local and superficial. A relatively greater or smaller area of the scheme may have to be reconstructed, down to a greater or less local depth ; but the main system, the fundamental belief in an objective world and all the chief elements and factors which enter into this, including above all the underlying belief in the objective status of perception as such—all this is never shaken. On the contrary, we have seen that it is further and most powerfully strengthened precisely by these impacts, and by everything we find to be involved in them, or demanded from us in order to cope with them.

It is essential to keep constantly in mind this primary division, renewed at each instant, between our purely subjective thoughts and beliefs and the new perceptual experience, impinging on us with an ungainsayable independence and outsideness, with which they find themselves confronted. But just because this happens at each moment and has been so happening all our lives, it is equally true that most of the content and structure of what are now " merely " our beliefs has been provided by the one-time *new perceptual experiences of the past*. They represent that experience (in every sense this time of " represent "), and indeed what the new perceptual content of each instant brings into operation is a set of beliefs based on those analogous *past " new "* perceptual experiences which have established a regular and apparently dependable pattern. Obviously, if we take the process back far enough, it becomes increasingly fallible because of the initial narrowness of the child's experience and his proneness to jump to conclusions ; whilst, again, in unfamiliar contexts or under certain special conditions adults may very readily fall into similar errors. But, subject always to progressive correction by further new perceptual material, it remains true that the main tenor of our beliefs about each separate kind of perceptual object (or other entity) has been furnished by earlier data of the same kind.

[1] We can, strictly speaking, go further still and emphasise, in precisely the same way, that in so far as our beliefs posit the *continuance* of our perceptual field, in part or as a whole, every moment of actual experienced continuance is a new confirmatory test, since each such moment *could* bring a change (slight or considerable or radical), and some moments, however small a *proportion*, do in fact bring unexpected ones.

Thus the correct picture is that if we take a cross-section of our psychic history at any time, we have on the one side the new experience which is actually in course of happening and on the other all the products or outcomes of our past experience which are functionally operative or specially revived in our thought as the new happening comes to us. From this comprehensive point of view, it must of course be borne in mind that the new happening includes new affective-conative and active experiences as much as perceptual ones, just as the retained past happening has done ; but the perceptual ones stand out in all the ways we have described, and above all in their relation to the scheme of anticipations (equally perceptual) which is projected in readiness for them. And by the same token on the side of our pre-existing psychic life and its contents there stands out the system of memories and beliefs embodying our past perceptual experience, or directly or indirectly derived from this.

On that side indeed the pattern is usually much more complicated than on that of our new experience, because of the many different forms of derivative products of our past history. Thus our scheme of beliefs about the perceptual world goes vastly beyond the scope of our own direct experience (including the whole of the inferential work we do on this), because of all the social information which gets grafted on our individual learning. And over and above everything in our beliefs which has good claims to be regarded as authentic knowledge about the objective order of things, we have a great domain of less assured opinions, theories, ideas and conjectures passing more or less continuously into avowed imaginings and fantasies, but for the most part clearly deriving their content, in one way or another, from that of perceptual experience, just like our system of authenticated information. However, these complexities do little to detract from our broad sense of the distinctness and uniqueness of the system, firstly, of our actual memories of the perceptual experiences which have happened to us, and secondly of the social information, historical and scientific, about the objective world which we know to rest upon fully tested and established perceptual evidence. In particular the distinction between fantasy and what we call " fact ", i.e., the beliefs which we rely upon as true to fact, is one about which in principle—and in an overwhelming majority of cases, in practice—we are perfectly clear and on which indeed the whole direction and control of our lives, moment by moment, depends.

We have of course our difficulties in keeping the *borders* of the two psychic domains distinct and particularly in preventing local intrusions from that of fantasy into that of " fact " ; at the best, as we have seen, numerous graduated passages from one to the other are provided by an endless variety of speculations, suppositions, hunches, intuitions, etc., of every degree of probability and improbability. But we do our utmost to preserve and apply at all times the main division, and even to keep the intermediate formations stamped as intermediate, and by and large we are successful —and thus alone preserve ourselves and carry most of our everyday activities through to their intended issue. What the descriptive analysis of this section has sought to show is precisely the cumulative structure of distinctions and demarcations by which we are enabled to achieve so effectively a division which is so essential to us : the segregation of our system of (mainly) trustworthy beliefs about the world of " fact " from all the rest of our psychic life. For this means not only from all our feelings and wishes and needs and fears, but also from all the work or play of our fantasy, as under the influence (and often the pressure) of one impulse or another it re-directs or re-shapes, breaks up and re-combines the elements of our past experiences in its own countless different ways.

(19) The foregoing leads us to a final note about the margins and limits of the solid structure of cumulatively verified beliefs which we have described.

(i) First of all we should bring into our story, however summarily, those various familiar types of experience (already alluded to earlier) which can so readily appear, or be made to appear, as stumbling-blocks in the way of any simple-minded common sense belief in a " given," objective world. These experiences range from mirror images or other reflections and shadows to refraction effects, optical illusions, mirages, perceptual anomalies of the most diverse kinds, dreams, hallucinations and delusions. They can plausibly be marshalled in such wise as to seem to blur almost completely the distinction between what is subjective and what is objective, and so to leave no logical foundation for our naïve faith in our " real " world.

Yet the plain fact is that it does not in the least work out that way. In philosophic debate, within the circle of ideas and procedures in which this usually moves, there is rarely much opportunity of bringing to bear the relevant full psychological evidence ; but in practice we have no difficulty—as the very existence of the above concepts show—in distinguishing between each of these special classes of experience and that of genuine veridical perception. Most of us have our occasional lapses ; only, we know how to correct these. The child has to learn gradually to acknowledge each separate category in its own right, and then to allow for it. In effect, he has no serious trouble in doing so. His picture of the objective world develops a degree of cohesion and solidity and consistency which keeps all apparent anomalies marginal and permits him to fit most of them in eventually as only special local cases.

Our working criterion for segregating out the misleading and pseudo-perceptions from the authentic ones is in truth precisely that of their non-cohesion with the stable and progressive system of the latter. In the simplest kinds of cases, such as those of mirror images or of bent-looking sticks in water, the child merely discovers himself in the presence of unwarranted anticipations, which are in fact falsified and thus corrected. Taking his experiences at their apparent perceptual face-value, he expects to find the seen object palpably and solidly (with all the other appropriate " object " properties) behind the mirror, or to encounter an actual bent stick when the latter is pulled out of the water or touched whilst in it. Now not only does he find nothing corresponding to these expectations, but quite a lot of *further* experiences help to isolate, discredit and destroy them. The mirror image is not only extraordinarily like a particular thing in *front* of the mirror, but moves and changes with this, can be produced and removed at will by means of the object in front, etc., etc. And it joins up with a class of similar experiences of " reflections " which each of them have their own parallel anomalous features, *in addition* to no corresponding object being ever found present. So that in the end the child builds up the new notion of a property belonging to certain kinds of surface of reproducing the mere visual likeness of objects in front of them, without any further thought of actual objects behind or underneath them. In the same sort of way, the bent-looking stick is not only not found bent when taken out of the water, but also if completely immersed it ceases to look bent ; the point of apparent bending can be made to change at will ; the same kind of thing can be done with other sticks and other objects, and so on. So that again the child can presently replace his first falsified assumption by the new idea of a special characteristic of *water* of producing the visual appearance of bentness in objects only partly placed in it. This is then duly further confirmed by his discovering or learning that the same characteristic applies (in varying degrees) to other liquids and, if he pursues his inquiries, going on to relate it to the passage of light generally through different media.

Comparable processes occur in connection with the other types of experience enumerated above. There is first of all a local breakdown of expectation (the *seemingly* shorter of two lines in certain optical illusions proves *on measurement* to be exactly the same, etc. ; or the appearance of a pool of water dissolves when its apparent location is approached) ; whilst later on there is a concourse of further features of the misleading kind of experience, and of its distinctive setting or occasion, which place it apart and build up round it a *new* expectation-scheme based on its established lack of objective reality. This comes to apply for most of us even to dreams and momentary hallucinations, which whilst they last have a convincingness all their own. In particular, as regards dreams, the child soon notes how presently they break off or dissolve in clear disjunction from all the stable and cumulative rest of his perception-and-belief system, and how in fact they only occur in certain characteristic and limited situations of his own, which can themselves be defined beforehand, and which usually rule out the very possibility of the dreamt activities and perceptions being objectively real or veridical. The case of momentary hallucinations generally falls into place in a similar way.

Thus, as we have said, each of these kinds of experience settles down eventually in its distinctive class, itself capable of being turned into a subject for attention and for cumulative learning and knowledge. They become types of *psychological* happenings which we study in their own right, without being disturbed or misled by them. We recognise indeed that they, or some of them, remain apt to take us in temporarily (even mirrors can continue to do so if deliberately arranged to deceive, or if some chance has suitably placed them) ; but we can point to plenty of other situations and occasions which are specially conducive to error, and the way to correction of such errors is no more difficult for us in the former class of cases than in any other. And if some of us are so carried away by particular types of these experiences that we become incapable of resisting them and making the requisite corrections, that again is the kind of exception which illuminates and further supports its rule. Habitual proneness to hallucinations and still more to delusions is recognised by us as a disturbance of the reality sense and symptom of mental derangement. And where this proneness is marked, there goes with it a characteristic further set of facts : the person's system of adaptive action breaks down in greater or less degree, and often indeed wholly ; he becomes incapable of " looking after himself " or unfit to be allowed to act freely, etc., etc. His dominant scheme of beliefs may prove itself delusive in the fullest sense by cutting him off in every way from our common objective reality.

(ii) When all this has been established, however, it must be accepted, and on the present empirical and historical approach to knowledge perhaps more clearly than on any other, that there can be no ultimate certainty about even the most strongly buttressed and firmly secured reading of our experience (so far). In particular, hallucinations, delusions and perhaps still more in the end what remains the oddest part of our experience-history, the self-segregated world of dreams, leave over an ultimate question. We can have no final answer to the fear which occasionally invades most of us that, for anything we can really prove to the contrary, we may be the victims of hallucinations ourselves, collectively as well as individually, and above all of some single enduring hallucination or larger dream which forms our entire world-picture : one from which we may some time come to, in goodness knows what sort of authentic " real " world. But beyond admitting the irrefutable possibility inherent in this notion or speculative fantasy, we can do nothing with it ; the fact remains that even if we were living within such a wholesale hallucination or dream, we should still have all the overwhelming system of reasons already set out here for maintaining to the full our crucial scheme of distinctions between the objective and the subjective, the " real " and the (sub-) " dream " sides, within our supposed larger dream. And we should have both the same means and the same grounds as we do now for carefully segregating our local sub-hallucinations, sub-illusions, etc., from our far stabler and more coherent " objective " system of perception and action. Indeed, so long as our experience continued along its present lines, all our beliefs would have to remain as they are, just because their main foundation, the belief in an objective world, is no idle theory, but a system of representations not only of the present and the past but also, through this, of our own future (the future of our actual experiences) which this is continually testing and verifying. Naturally, if all the course of things, everything that befell us, suddenly started changing violently in all directions, we should have new food for thought (if we survived to do any thinking), and might have to begin all over again. However so far the one sustained refrain of all the vicissitudes and all the history of our experience remains that the more it changes, the more it is the same thing.

(20), (iii) By way of conclusion, we must glance at another and rather more practical set of qualifications, or potential qualifications, of our story. We have brought out the dominant and controlling part played by perceptual experience in our belief in and picture of the objective world. That is in accord with our ordinary common sense assumptions, and we have sought to show that it is the special status which perceptual experience establishes for itself (in all the ways we have described) which is the ultimate warrant for the above belief.

Yet it does not follow that perceptual experience, or for that matter any thought-structure directly elaborated from this, is our only source of knowledge of, or information about, the objective or real world existing independently of our states. There are admittedly many other claimants, and nothing that has been said so far is intended to prejudge their claims. We have only been concerned here with the part (far-reaching as we have shown it to be) played by our perceptual experience, without seeking to consider or assess any other factor or suggested factor. Innate or inherited knowledge, instinct, intuition, telepathy, clairvoyance, inspiration, revelation, mystic vision, veridical or prophetic dreaming, prophecy, pure logical reasoning, occult or magical powers, ethical, religious and aesthetic experience, etc., etc. : all these individually and in varying combinations have been put forward at times as sources of valid and often of overriding knowledge of the real world or " reality." Many of these sources are indeed widely thought at present to be fully established by evidence or reasoning which can withstand the most searching scrutiny. It would be a vast further enterprise, which cannot be contemplated here, to examine the grounds for each of these claims and to try to determine where and how they fit in, though in our last chapter we shall return to a very brief glance at their bearings, after our own main sketch has been completed. The only point which it seems legitimate to make at this stage is that the proper examination and appraisal of any and all these claims must obviously *take into account* the immense cumulative structure of assured and tested knowledge of which we have traced the outline, and by the same token the world-picture to which this leads.

That picture might have to be amplified or modified, but it cannot be disregarded or negated ; it must in the main be accepted as what is already established, if only because—as we have noted—it is being *re-tested and re-confirmed* in a myriad places and a myriad ways every moment, throughout the entire fabric not only of our individual lives and activities, but of our whole far-flung civilisation.

In actual fact most of the claims referred to above do accept or assume at least a large portion of our ordinary common-sense-perceptual world-picture, and indeed some of them invoke in their own support direct perceptual evidence or verification. Whether this is usually done with an adequate sense of what is involved is another question. But others among these claims are definitely set up as rival or superior ones, giving knowledge of some reality, or part or aspect of " reality," which is not accessible to any shape or form of perception, or is inherently incapable of being perceptually experienced, but which is nevertheless " real " or " objective " either in the same or (often) in a higher sense.

Once again, nothing that has been said here prejudges whether or not such claims are valid. However, it is not merely reasonable but essential to call upon those who propound them to specify first of all quite clearly the meaning which *they* assign to the terms " real " or " objective," and the criteria by which they distinguish " reality " or " objective existence " in *their* sense from " mere " feeling or thinking. The claims cannot be assessed until the nature of what they claim has been made plain. Few even among the advocates of the extremest forms of them are likely to dispute the phenomenological or psychological proposition that there is some difference in status between say fairy-tale fantasies and the statements in Bradshaw, the minutes of a meeting, or a description of a scientific experiment. Or, more generally, that there is much which we think and feel (from day-dreams to pains, discomforts, excitements and gratifications) which does not even *purport* to represent or reflect an objective reality that is outside of or independent of itself but that somehow corresponds to it or is revealed by it. Therefore if anything we think or feel is held to be in a different case from such admittedly purely subjective experiences or states, the first need is to define and establish the character of the believed difference and the criteria on which we judge that any particular set of thoughts or feelings belongs to that " different " class.

We have shown that there is no difficulty about this in all the

range of notions and beliefs which claim reference and correspondence to " objective " realities accessible through perceptual
experience (though where we are dealing with pre-scientific levels
of thought we must beware of beliefs that have some overlap with
the world of perceptual experience, but also go far beyond anything which the latter has in fact validated or is capable of validating). But where the reference is to " realities " or " objective
existences " which are by hypothesis outside the realm of " mere "
perception, we must, if we do not want merely to bemuse and
deceive ourselves, insist firmly on clear alternative specifications
of what is here *meant* by " reality " or " objective existence "
(what these signs or sounds are intended to convey)—and what
this meaning *has in common* with our ordinary usage of these
symbols to justify their employment and so the implied claim
to the connotation and status which they ordinarily carry. We
cannot be too much on our guard against the unconsidered transfer, through the mere use of the same symbol, of all the claims and
titles built up by the tremendous cumulative history of our perceptual experience *as* perceptual experience, to some other sort
of meaning or definition which may not have the least right to
them.

This issue cannot be pursued any further now. We must
return to our structure of unquestionably learnt and tested knowledge, based on just the above history, of which we have not as
yet traced anything like the full extent and strength. The next
chapter, in particular, about the experiential basis for our belief
in causality and in the objective causal system of our world constitutes an inseparable part of the story. These last paragraphs
have merely been concerned to make plain that the present
approach implies no advance denial of other sources of genuine
knowledge (that is, information of or about some existence or
reality independent of the mere psychic occurrence and content
of the thought or belief we regard as embodying such information).
But any claims on behalf of such believed sources must be adequately assessed on their own merits, and such assessment cannot
make sense if it merely *disregards* all the experiential knowledge
which is already clearly and overwhelmingly established.

CHAPTER VI

EXPERIENTIAL BASIS FOR OUR BELIEF IN CAUSALITY

(1) We have emphasised all along, firstly, that our experience-history is one, and all the main elements in its structure and organisation are interdependent, intersupporting and inter-developing, and secondly that there is a particularly close and integral relation between our belief in an objective world and our notion of causality. This has made inevitable a certain amount of anticipation of the ground to be covered in the present chapter, and we have in effect already built up the pattern of a thoroughly causal experience-world. Most significantly, the key-concept of " control " has come to occupy a more and more pivotal place in our story. However, we have yet to relate this concept more closely to our normal causal ideas and beliefs, and to bring together in a single whole all the chief experience-elements which express themselves in our distinctive notion of causality, over and above that of the objective world.

(2) We must begin by noting that whilst what we call common sense is broadly right in its way of conceiving and affirming the objective world, this is not equally true as regards causality. Here the position is that it has correctly taken in a vast number of separate causal lessons, both local and general, but has never integrated them into an organised whole which adequately re-flects and combines them. There are a number of fallacies and confusions about causal relations which are still widely held, even among educated people, and lead to the most far-reaching and fatal errors. Furthermore the situation is not made any better by the attempt, on the part of many scientists (following the lead of the empiricist philosophers), to cut through all the difficulties and entanglements supposed to be inherent in the common sense approach by defining causality as simply invariable succession. This substitutes a small and relatively unimportant fragment of the experience-content of our causal notions for the whole.

Common sense remains far nearer the mark ; all the essential components are present in the *sum* of its causal approaches to its world, and under favouring conditions most or all of the relevant ones may be combined in its attitude to some particular problem or field, just as they are *in practice* in the habitual procedures of scientists. On the other hand common sense also falls all too frequently into the fallacious assumption of " one " cause or " the " cause for any given fact or situation ; it gets into endless confusions between different kinds of causes and between causes, reasons and explanations ; and it is quite apt to apply the notion in contexts in which it does not make sense. What is needed, therefore, as a remedy for this state of affairs, is no new thesis but merely the *explicit assembly and integration* of all the major elements which common sense tends to acknowledge and utilise *separately* ; the result can then be seen not to clash with it, but on the contrary to take up and satisfy *all* its demands—in line, as we have said, with its own best concrete practice.

(3) As a preliminary to our own approach, we may turn back for a moment to the scientific or rather pseudo-scientific notion of invariable succession. This of course is intended to get rid of the supposed primitive and exploded idea of causal *action* or *efficacy*—and if necessary also to do without the supposed naïve metaphysical assumption of objects. We have already suggested, on the contrary, that objects, and moreover objects acting and acted upon, controlling and controlled, constitute the most central and irresistible finding of our experience *as experience*. To try to eliminate them and their actions and interactions is in effect just to emasculate our conception of causality ; and scientists themselves completely disprove—even as they disregard—the above nominal definition in every experiment they perform.

In our last chapter, we have shown that our experience of the *controlling status and operation* of the perceptual foci we come to acknowledge as objects is one of the major elements which enters into this acknowledgment, supports it and helps to form the meaning of the very notion of objects. What we have now to do is to survey more specifically our early experiences of (*a*) learning the ways in which our object-foci control us and act upon us (*b*) learning the ways in which we can counter-control them and act upon them (*c*) learning to watch and take in the ways in which they control and act upon one another. All this is then further combined with (*d*) our experiences of the ways in which successive happenings are linked with one another and, again, of the ways in which these apparent linkages sometimes fail (*e*) our learning to *seek*, in respect of any kind of happening or state which is of special interest to us, the key of some previous type of happening which controls it and either indicates, if it occurs, that the former is going to follow, or else can itself be made to occur and so used as a means of bringing the former about, and (*f*) our finding that this search always does lead, sooner or later, to such a key, and though these keys rarely prove infallible to begin with, that they can always be further amplified and improved until they reach an extremely high level of reliability. But (*d*), (*e*) and (*f*)usually lead back to (*c*), which in turn develops in close interrelation with (*a*) and (*b*). And it is crucial for the whole developing experience-complex that among the objects we learn earliest to acknowledge, there is our own body, existing just like others and in the same field (however peculiarly—and controllingly—it is also linked all the time with ourselves as experients), and more and more found to be in interaction with other objects and bodies, i.e., acted upon by them and acting on them, in precisely the same way as they interact with one another.

(4) Let us glance briefly again at each of these experience-groups.

(*a*), (i) Our first *clear* encounter with object-control emerges directly from our attentional activity—and passivity. A particular focus arrests us and holds us, and this very experience becomes the earliest coefficient of objectivity, the initial stage in the conversion of an experience-focus into experience *of* a focus. We are undergoing our first pointed experience of being controlled, and this marks the beginning of our whole future cognitive development. Attending to object-foci and letting ourselves be controlled by them in various ways is the road by which we learn most of what we eventually know about them ; and if we go astray in the anticipations we form about their characters, the process of suffering their control again and being forcibly corrected by them is that by which our expectations about them, or pictures of them, are eventually made right.

(ii) Even earlier than this order of experience of object-control there is that fundamental other which takes a little longer to become plain but then proves even more vital to the child : there is a focus of control outside his feelings and wantings and strivings on which his states of satisfaction and non-satisfaction, pleasure and pain, comfort and distress depend. Something has to intervene—and can be seen and heard and in all other ways perceived as intervening—if his cravings are to be turned into gratifications, and his discomforts, distresses and fears relieved. This something *is* constantly intervening, but also often fails to do so, however urgently craved for. And often also it withdraws itself, in the same all-too-perceptible fashion, whereupon the child's state is suddenly changed again, too often back to painfulness and all sorts of other feelings he wants to struggle away from. Furthermore that particular perceptual focus, which more and more takes shape as the *object*-focus, the *object*, the *person* the child learns to acknowledge as his mother, very often exerts its all-powerful controlling action in conjunction with other perceptual object-foci, by being seen acting on them, removing them, or bringing them, or operating with them. Other objects more or less like the mother intervene in comparable ways, directly and in conjunction with ancillary agencies.

The child undergoes in these ways, under the most palpable control of those objects and their witnessed activities, the experiences of being nursed and tended, lifted, carried, rocked, clothed and unclothed, washed and cleansed, etc., etc. All this joins up into one consistent and connected story : the perceptual agencies round him, coming and going and acting and being acted upon, change and control his states and his experiences, from the most important to the least so, in a hundred successive ways. That happens every day, and through endless repetitions with variations, he has the opportunity of sorting out the master control, the other major ones, and the mere instruments and means, as well as the main pattern of the relations between them. And as he develops a more and more clear and distinctive awareness of that further object which presently becomes the most central of all for his consciousness, his own body, and its peculiar relation to his experiences, he learns to link up at the same time the control exercised by the intervening objects over his feeling-states with their action, direct and indirect, and both witnessed and felt, on his body.

(*b*) At the same time as the child learns these lessons of undergoing, i.e., suffering control and action upon himself (both pleasant and unpleasant), he is also picking up his first experiences and lessons of exercising control and effective action himself.

We have seen that there is one early mode which proves to be very potent but quite soon turns into a blind alley, and can become an aberration into permanent error. This is the activity of crying, which strongly tends to bring the chief power-wielding presence to the child. For most practical purposes, however, it is gradually discarded in favour of procedures more directly related to the specific situation, though it may leave traces which confuse the later notion of causality, even if it does not lead straight on to a world of archaic animistic or anthropomorphic beliefs.

But there are at least two other ways of action and control duly discovered by the child, which open up to him avenues of genuine and cumulative progress.

For the first, we can go as far back as his early random movements of his hands and feet, which soon call perceptual attention to themselves and may at any time bring about further perceptual happenings. Presently the infant makes the vital discovery that by repeating the movement or activity he can renew the rest of the experience, and if it is something at all dramatic, he will thereupon practise it on and on with the utmost energy and gusto. When he thus finds his way (with adult help) to real noise-making, rattling, banging, etc., he obviously feels himself on top of the world, and his repertory soon expands further to pushing, pulling, lifting and dropping, tearing and bursting, and manipulating every sort of thing or toy that will give a good lusty reward and so a real sense of something done, of an authentic, resounding effect achieved. These processes then expand and develop into the whole world of play and into all the skills and powers and modes of effective controlling action the child thus learns.

Secondly, over and above the early activities which he enjoys as energising and effect-producing for their own sake, he soon picks up the first beginnings of actions which directly serve to influence or control his own affective states in ways similar to those practised by his mother or other persons round him. He learns for himself to relieve pressures by moving clothes, etc. ; to draw wanted objects to him ; to co-operate in more and more of the processes applied to him, and so on. In other words, he starts on the great high road of purposive activity, exercising control on and through things in order to secure his own aims, using them as means and instruments, and becoming a more and more conscious and deliberate and powerful causal agent in his own right.

(c) And naturally his progress in this direction owes a great deal to yet another line of concurrent development, which in the end leads the child much further still and can indeed carry him as far as the full world of scientific inquiry and understanding. From his first few months onward he gradually learns to make use of his opportunities of witnessing and watching the actions of objects on one another—first of all in direct terms of his mother's and other persons' ministrations to him, or their other most obvious operations round him, but before long with a wider range. He pays increasing attention to *all* the goings on within his perceptual field, and as his own effect-producing activities expand, he will seek to include among them some of those he has watched, and will practise them and watch them turn by turn. Others of course will be beyond his scope, but in that case he may become all the more interested in getting to know all about them, if only in the hope that he may thus be enabled eventually to participate in them. And all the time, as he learns to pay attention to the most diverse kinds of processes and happenings and changes taking place around him, his sense of the causal relations and interconnections of things is being enlarged and enriched, as well as confirmed and consolidated. The ticking and striking of a clock, running water, striking of matches, switching on of lights, the rain or snow outside, the burning of a fire, the dissolving of sugar in milk or tea, a draught blowing out a candle or making a curtain flutter, clothes being washed, dried and ironed, and a thousand similar and different occurrences go on building up in the child the sense of objects acting, being acted upon and interacting, being changed and controlled and exercising their own control. This theme is then taken up on a larger and larger scale in the wider world round the child, in the streets and the fields, in shops and workshops, railway stations and great factories, on the banks of rivers and on the seas.

It is obvious that the above several modes of causal experience, of being controlled, controlling, and learning to know the mutual controlling activities of other objects, will tend to support and reinforce and develop one another, and thus, under favourable conditions, will more and more merge in a single cumulative broad movement of advance. We need not do more here than to show the process (nourished from its threefold but intercommunicating roots) started on its way, since its further course lies open to anyone who wishes to follow it. The main lead is no doubt taken in the earlier stages of the history both of the race and the individual by the endeavour to secure sufficient powers of control to ward off or counteract those ways of being controlled which are painful to us, and to secure the positive aims which, from occasion to occasion, we set ourselves. Thus we collect an immense amount of practical causal knowledge about the properties and powers of things, for direct good or ill (our good or ill), or for their use as tools and instruments for acting on other things ; and even if we do not go on to any generalised scientific causal interest pursued for its own sake, we do tend to *learn*, at least in selected practical fields, the most pregnant of our causal lessons. If we are in difficulties or find ourselves stopped on the way to some purpose, our one hope of an answer always lies in trying to find further causal or controlling relationships which will overcome the obstacle or bridge the gap : our belief in causality is our most sure key to the knowledge which is power.

(5), (*d*) Yet all the foregoing, though it gives us the final hard core of our future sense of causality, is still no more than one section (even though the central one) of the structure of our complete causal notion. We have yet to bring in the whole of the temporal factor, with its far-reaching implications. In the limited form usually contemplated by the philosophic-pseudo-scientific tradition, the temporal aspect of causality would only provide a further and very minor fragment of the story ; but in its proper vital interrelation with the rest, it immensely broadens our perspective and brings us straight on to the highway leading to the full scientific causal picture of our world. In particular it helps more than anything else to shift the stress away from the primary ego-centrism which tends to confine our interest to the powers of control we need for our own aims—that is, the avoidance of disagreeable and the achievement of desired states of affairs. For in this way beyond any other we are forced to learn the vital importance, even to our own aims, of watching and following out the interactions and interrelations of things *among themselves*, i.e. irrespective of their immediate bearings on us.

What we are concerned with here, once more, is our attention to the course of objective *events*, the expectations this leads us to form and the history of those expectations. But it is essential to stress again that this is *not* merely a matter of sensation A being followed by sensation B, or even of unit-event A being followed by unit-event B, and our thus learning to expect B from A ; and if the succession occurs regularly enough, calling B " caused " by A, or anyway causally associated with A. The events are complex happenings or changes in a broad field, merely *selected for attention* from a continuum of such changes, and perceived as happening to at least one complex object, but more often as involving two or more. Furthermore, the expectations which, to begin with, are formed if a specific sequence or train of events is frequently repeated, or impresses itself very vividly, are mostly falsified sooner or later, whereupon however (if the conditions are not too unfavourable), they are not given up, but subjected to vital processes of readjustment which may affect not only the immediate expectation but our view of the whole background and even the general processes by which we form expectations at large.

What the child has to become habituated to is in effect no simple world of settled objects mostly quiescent but with just a limited capacity for acting and being acted upon. What actually confronts him is an endless flow of happenings, largely cyclical, with a host of lesser and greater cycles superimposed on one another (and to be only slowly learnt), but including also day by day and month by month a certain proportion of *new* kinds of events. Many of these in turn recur (though some of them only at irregular intervals), and they thus become recognition-objects in their own right, and, by the same token, stimuli and foci for expectation systems. Thus there impresses itself on the child the fact that one kind of these irregular, intrusive happenings often ushers in some further one of quite a distinct kind (i.e. distinct enough not to be treated as part of a single event), so that as soon as he recognises the first, this acts as a signal to him to expect the second. On that basis he builds up, as we have seen, a successful scheme of pre-adaptation and appropriate anticipative action, up to the limiting case of actively intervening, to try to *prevent* the further expected happening. But presently the sequence fails him, with all the accompaniments and results we have already worked out. And then it becomes extremely important for him to be able to distinguish the instances where the expectation will not fail him from those where it may or will.

Nor is this all. Even if he comes to foresee, with dependable correctness, what one of these intrusive happenings will bring in its train, that may not give him time enough to deal satisfactorily with its sequels ; or for that matter it may have an immediate undesired impact on him ; or, on the other hand, it may have a very welcome impact on him, which he wants to repeat, but does not know how to. Each of these cases in its specific way makes the child want to foresee even the *earlier* happening, and so to know whether there is in turn any previous occurrence which will serve as an advance signal of the second link in the chain. Or still better, whether there is any previous occurrence which will not only definitely bring the one in issue *in its train*, but which can perhaps itself be either brought about or stopped by his own action, thus giving him control over what is to follow.

It is clear that all this is continuous with the efforts we have already noted on the part of the child to build up his own more and more comprehensive and adequate equipment of control. But it has also its own distinctive sphere just because he is concerned the whole time not only with a world of continuing and more or less stable objects, but also with one of endless successive happenings which he must try to learn to know correctly no less than the order of objects, i.e. in which he must try to learn to foresee as much as possible, as early as possible and as truly or reliably as possible. Thus he has to develop a special timewise attention and type of learning, from given events both forward to what they bring in their train and backward to what has brought them in its train. And this, as we have noted, applies above all to new, intrusive and irregular happenings, as distinct from all the regular cyclical routines ; to these he soon becomes accustomed and, because of their very regularity, they come to form the barely regarded framework of his life.

In the outcome we get two types of interest ; according as, on the one hand, something is already known about the time-sequence, but we need a more and more specific selection and determination of the set of happenings which can be *depended* upon to lead to or bring about a given other ; or, on the other hand, we are confronted with an event about the antecedents of which we know nothing, and we therefore attempt to discover what it is that in fact leads to or brings about that kind of event.

(6), (*e*) and (*f*) Chiefly in the foregoing way, but with help also from the directions adumbrated before, the child is carried on to the full conscious crystallisation of his causal experiences in the *causal question*. This he expresses unambiguously in the forms " What makes . . . " and " What made . . . " and more ambiguously in some though not all of his questions " why." The latter form in all its implications will occupy us more fully in the next chapter. But the causal question, however expressed, marks the stage of a developed and deliberate demand for causal information. The child knows now that this is generally available. He has definitely laid hold of the idea of the control or determination of any happening or finding that provokes his interest by some particular X, with which he himself is not familiar (yet), but which can always be provided by those who have enough knowledge. And the causal question addressed to others leads of course, in the final stage of first hand scientific inquiry, to the same question addressed to the subject himself and ushering in actual scientific investigation.

In the earlier phase of the child's social quest for causal information, the unintegrated variety of his own causal experiences leads to an equal variety of potential meanings of his questions, all closely related and capable of integration even if only rarely receiving it. He may be wanting to find out the particular antecedents of a particular event or state, or the general controlling antecedent of a particular *kind* of event or state ; or he may desire to know what controls a given property or characteristic or way of behaviour ; or he may wish to understand what controls or determines some *difference* of character or behaviour of apparently *similar* things, or some difference of outcome of apparently similar occurrences. Or he may draw on all his experience of happenings which were about to take place, but did not because something (or somebody) had intervened to stop them (counter-controlled them), and he may want to ascertain in a given case whether something had not similarly intervened to prevent a particular occurrence, and if so, what it was.

The medley of causal experiences of the most diverse kind in the child's mind is made very much worse by the large special class which gets built up round human actions and products, and to some extent also round those of other living things. He learns more and more that in this order of instance the controlling factor is a peculiar kind of cause in the human or living agent—the type of cause which in its most developed human form we call a motive or intention or aim or purpose and which goes beyond the immediate effect and relates this to human desires and feelings. That is a kind of controlling cause so ubiquitous around the child in his early days, and so naturally coming home to himself and fitting in with all his own nisus, that there is a marked tendency for him to look first of all for a cause of the same kind for almost everything *of an assimilable type* that arouses the causal quest in him. This tendency he expresses in a great many of his " why's " ; but that it is not by any means universal is shown by his free use also of the form " What makes . . . " or " What made . . . " (to be carefully distinguished from the quite different question : "Who made . . . "). And of course in its own proper field, viz. the large one of human actions and products, the search for controlling psychological causes, of the class of motives and purposes, is for the most part as legitimate as the quest for physical ones is elsewhere. Outside their legitimate domain, most of the demands for motives and purposes gradually wither away.

(7) If now we try to reduce the common sense medley to order, still taking account of all the different but interrelated kinds of actual " *causal* " experiences, but of such experiences only, we may first distinguish and then combine the following components :

(i) *The Active or Operative Core*

A myriad of the most diverse experiences lead us to expect, or believe, that for every kind of happening or change (whether viewed as such, or approached in terms of its end-state or product), there is a specific type of previous occurrence which has brought it about, or whenever this occurrence takes place, *tends* to bring it about. And the core of the previous occurrence is almost if not quite invariably either the arrival or the introduction of a new agency or factor within the local field, or (closely allied to this), an alteration or increase of an existing agency or factor in it. (The " local field " may consist of a single body undergoing the mechanical impact of another body ; of a quantity of material to which is added a quantity of other material reacting chemically with it ; of the estuary of a river receiving a tidal wave, etc., etc. The size of the relevant " field " may vary from the microscopic to the astronomic. The point is the new introduction of *something*—great or small, a new major force or substance, or the slightest application of a finger to a trigger or a switch—which was previously extraneous to the " field." The introduction is usually by actual spatial motion either into the field, or anyway into its margin of influenceability.)

This generalised expectation is continually strengthened and consolidated because it is constantly confirmed not only in cases where we have already *established* a specific linkage, but also in all those where we are thus led to look for a still unknown one—and to find it.

(ii) *The Qualifying and Limiting Penumbra*

But the expectation is also confirmed and consolidated, at the same time as qualified and extended, by numerous experiences where it appears at first to have broken down. If a specific effect is present, we can often safely infer a specific cause ; yet if the cause is present, we learn to say only that it will *tend* to produce the effect. What happens is that where the latter does not come about, we find that we have thought of our causal relation in too simple a form. We do not have to give it up, but we have to introduce further co-controlling factors. And they can always be found, and the causal relation then formulated in a more dependable form.

We gradually learn in fact that a whole hierarchy of co-controlling factors has always to be present if there is to be full assurance of the effect being produced. A comprehensive series of *conditions* has to be fulfilled. Some of them merely specify more

E

closely the character of the causal agency or the mode of its introduction. Others bear in a parallel way on the character of the
field. These latter lead on to still others specifying earlier causal
factors which must already have been at work before a given
immediate causal agency can bring about a particular result :
preparatory circumstances, predisposing ones, etc. Again, there
may be a wide range of broad general permissive conditions without which the effect has been found to fail.

All these are matters of experience, of trial and error. We can
never be sure that we have allowed for everything that is relevant.
Over and over again we discover the relevance of some variable
only when we find that our effect has failed us and then track
down a change in a factor which had hitherto happened to be
constant or had not varied sufficiently or appropriately and which
therefore we had taken for granted. Usually, once we have the
cue, we can verify and establish a new regular rule of causal
relevance, so that the principle of causality is not in the least
brought into question, but merely the particular case more
adequately understood and formulated.

(iii) *Interfering, Deflecting or Preventing "Causes"*

Yet another class of cases where apparent exceptions merely
serve to vindicate and strengthen the rule is where our expectation
breaks down, but closer inquiry shows that some other causal
agency was also operating in or on the same field, in such a way
as to counteract or at least deflect or modify the ordinary result
of the agency on which we based our original expectation.

There is obviously no hard and fast division between this class
of cases and the factors in our previous group ; we can indeed
say, if we wish, that the conditions which must be fulfilled before
any given agency can be relied upon to produce its characteristic
effect must always include the absence of counteracting or preventing or deflecting " causes. " Nevertheless, the demonstrated
presence of a previously unsuspected counteracting cause is so
striking and frequent an illustration of the way in which our
common sense notion of active or operative causality is in the end
re-confirmed by the very facts that seem to throw doubt on it,
that it merits its own clear emphasis.

(8), (iv) *Reciprocal Action of " Cause " and " Effect "*

If by " cause " we merely meant an *event* invariably anteceding
some other event, there could manifestly be no question of the
former being modified by the latter. But, as we have already
seen, we mean vastly more, and most typically the introduction

into a field of a new agency, which then operates on or in that field according to its own character and brings about an appropriate change in it. This, however, must sooner or later raise the question : what of the action, or reaction, of the field on the introduced agency ?

Very often indeed there is none, or rather none that is visible to us or of interest to us, and in such cases this fact plus our angle of approach usually lead us to focus exclusively on the introduced agency as our central causal factor. The further result then is that we tend very commonly just to think of the agency in question as " the cause " of the effect produced, without paying any more attention to the obvious fact that it is not its existence but its having been *newly brought to bear* which has started off the effect at a particular time and place. Thus our thought is deflected from any counter-effect which may be produced on our agency by its new field of application, and, as we have said, in many cases this does not matter because in truth it remains substantially unchanged, and may indeed go on producing the same kind of effect in the same unchanged way in an almost indefinite succession of new " fields."

The deflection of our thought is carried still further when, having split off our substantial causal agency from the *event* of its introduction into a given field, we decide, for a change, to place the whole stress on the latter aspect, and call this event " the " cause. We are also led in the same direction by all the cases of physical agencies which are already present in some field or situation without affecting it, but are then " started off " by a new minor occurrence. The latter may then easily be picked upon as the real causal fact, and from attending to the way in which only changes bring about changes, we may readily be brought to a pure " event " view of causality, which can seem very plausible but in fact, as we have said, treats a small fractional aspect as if it were the whole.

For the true position is that in most if not all causal sequences there is involved, besides the initiating new happening, the character of some substantive agency which either remains in existence during the sequence, or had previously had, or might in suitable circumstances have, continuing existence. In all such cases we learn more and more that what is set going is not necessarily only a one-way action of the agency on the field, but most often an interaction between them, in which the agency *suffers* some degree of change, as well as *produces* or *induces* it. In many instances, indeed, this is so manifest that we tend to view them from the start as a class apart, which later we expressly call inter-actions—the extreme type of case being the vast range of chemical phenomena where the bringing together of two or more sub-stances leads to both or all disappearing and a third, or a new set, being formed. But what is increasingly borne in on us is that even where the causal agency appears to retain its own character, and all our attention is focused on the effects " it " produces, that is rarely (if ever) the whole story. It is exposed to the action of its new field just as much as conversely, and *may* in turn undergo any and every degree of modification (down, at any rate, to near-zero). Furthermore the changes which it produces in the field may in turn react on it, sometimes in a limited, self-balancing cycle, sometimes in a cumulative progression. The important point which we have to recognise is that *interaction* is the inherent and basic pattern of causality, whilst the cases where the predomi-nant factor is or appears to be completely unaffected by the causal situation represent a restricted special class.

(v) *Negative Causality*

We are forced to attend to yet another aspect of our causal experiences and to learn to expand and develop this, when it is brought home to us to what an extent happenings both to us and around us are due not to the positive operations of particular agencies but to their cessation or removal. In a rudimentary form, of course, this is part and parcel of our first experiences both of being controlled and of learning to control (as well as of watching the actions and cessation of action of things around us). Our whole idea of operative causes carries with it as a counterpart the notion of their action stopping if they are removed, or in turn suitably acted upon, and the stoppage (and all its further con-sequences) is the happening we must often learn to aim at. (Or sometimes also to try to learn to prevent.)

But we have to go further and to free the above notion from its mere " counterpart " status and set it up in its own right. The cases that compel us to do so are all those where we were in the habit of taking the operation of some casual agency for granted, i.e. where we were not distinctively aware of this at all, but regarded it as a part of the nature, either of a particular scheme of things, or of our world at large. In such instances it is only the departure or removal (or sufficient weakening or diminution) of the agency which renders us alive to its contribution. Or rather, most often, an unexpected and usually disconcerting new series of happenings or changes sets us looking disturbedly for what has gone wrong ; and we then discover that the case is not one of some untoward new factor arriving or being introduced into our familiar field, but of something which we had hitherto regarded as a matter of course and paid no attention to, or not even been conscious of, having stopped or having been withdrawn.

It is interesting to note that in such situations we are clearly compelled to treat the *event* of the stoppage or withdrawal, and not the agency itself, as the cause of the effect which concerns us ; although it is obvious that the way in which it operated while it did (i.e., its nature and characteristic properties) was just as important and just as much the true causal factor as in all our positive cases. And of course in addition we are led at once to seek in turn for the *cause* of the stoppage or withdrawal—in the shape of any further factor or agency which has newly come into operation and of which the characteristic properties and action have had this particular effect.

Negative causality of the above kind, besides all its confirmations and consolidation of our positive notion, has a special significance, as we shall see, as a contributory to the unfolding of the next major component in our total causal scheme.

(vi) *Static or Passive Causality—Dependence and Interdependence*

A fundamental further development implicit in the processes of growth we have already sketched but carrying these farther away than ever from the naïve pseudo-scientific concept of invariable successions of *events* is the emergence of the notions first of dependence and then of interdependence. These are clearly already present in their main practical impoit as soon as we are forced to qualify our first simple assumptions of this or that agency *always* producing this or that effect, or this or that happening *always* bringing about such and such another. We find, through one falsified expectation after another, that it does not work out so, and we are compelled to attend to one factor after another which must *also* be there or right if our casual agency or event is to yield its due effect ; that is to say, on which the production of that effect *depends*.

The same sort of lesson, and the same resulting idea, emerge from all our experiences of negative causality of the type we have described above. They, as we have seen, establish *retrospectively* that a previous apparently settled and constant state of affairs *depended* on the continued presence and operation of some particular agency. Thus we become increasingly alive to the fact that as new happenings arise from previous new happenings, so the *absence* of these, the *maintenance* of a given state of affairs, depends on the maintenance, without any new happenings, of the causal factors which sustain it, or on which it depends.

In these ways we get the beginnings of a static-causal picture first of this and that local section and then of larger and larger portions of our world, till we learn to apply the same view to the whole. If any state, on whatever scale, continues, a large number of factors and conditions are involved in its maintenance and continuance. A disturbance of any of them may reveal its contribution ; any change in the state may prove to be due to such a disturbance rather than to the positive action of any new factor intervening (there may have been one further back to cause the upset—but this *may* be a great way back : the trouble may have been working up for a long time in the history of the agency in question).

Our developing static-causal approach is important just because we increasingly discover that continuing states are not an exception or one limited class of cases among others, but the general and pervasive rule. The notion is obviously a relative one, and we get limited persistence of local states in every degree, but this is not all. Even in changing states, there is a large element of continuance, and we find in fact that there is always a wider surrounding state which substantially goes on, and against which, or in terms of which, our very changes are measured. Persistence thus tends to present itself as, at least to all appearance, the most fundamental fact.

Yet our growing static-causal experiences and insight do not allow us to regard any particular continuing state or order of things, on however cosmic a scale, as necessarily the last word. Behind each successive larger persisting state we have always found once more sustaining and conditioning factors which were capable of suffering variation ; and sooner or later mutability has always again been brought home to us by the discovery of some happening or change which in fact arose from some variation in an apparently stable sustaining factor or condition.

On each such occasion it remains true that more survives than changes, else we should not even be able to describe the change. But each time we are forced to become more fully aware of all the invisible, static causality, both operative and conditioning, which provides the framework within which all our local visible causality works. And whilst if we look at only one particular order or area of fact, what is impressed upon us is its multiple dependences, attention to any wider range or area inevitably expands this notion to that of pervasive *inter*dependence. We are more and more led to think in terms of a system or scheme in which every part rests on the concurrence of the others, and in turn plays its own concurrent role ; an event or change anywhere brings about a whole cycle of other events or changes, and enforces a greater or lesser series of readjustments in a wide portion of the entire system before this achieves stable balance again. Actually events and changes are always going on, and as far as we can see, follow a vast number of at least partly distinct courses, which continually intersect and interact and generate yet further specific disturbances ; so that full equilibrium and stability are in fact never reached. But more or less distinct local systems or schemes (of all degrees of breadth) can be seen in at least temporary, more or less self-contained equilibrium ; can be seen suffering irruptive disturbances ; can be seen undergoing complex and widespread processes of change and readjustment ; and can be seen reaching again at length a state of equilibrium, or apparent equilibrium, even though often one that differs in far-reaching ways from the previous state.

(9), (vii) *Distinction Between Functional-structural and Historical Causality*

We have repeatedly approached the verge of a distinction, indeed a virtual bifurcation, in our causal approach to our world, which is almost wholly blurred in our ordinary common sense picture but is inherent in its experiential foundations and can readily be laid bare.

In a very large part both of our practical and of our cognitive dealings with our world we are concerned with *classes* of objects and their properties (controlling and controllable or usable), *classes* of events and their causes and effects, *classes* of processes and states and situations, and what they depend upon. It is because such classes of similar objects, etc., exist—and exist on all levels of similarity, so that they can be marshalled in comprehensive hierarchic systems—that we can build up bodies of cumulative knowledge and convert these into successful action and successful planning. We do so primarily in virtue of the transferability (subject to adjustment and correction) of our experience and of what we learn from this to each new member of each class which we meet ; and therefore what we mainly seek always is such *transferable* experience, learning and knowledge.

Yet that is far from universally true. There is also a realm of non-transferable individual knowledge which is of the utmost importance to us. (i) First of all, there are individual entities which are immensely significant to us as individuals, and about which we have to accumulate all the learning and understanding we can. This group includes our first most important external object (the mother), quite a number of subsequent personal objects, and also that unique quasi-external one which, by and large, remains the most momentous single thing for each of us throughout our life, our body. (ii) In our concrete experience we are in fact always confronted with individual objects, events, etc., and we are forced to learn that these mostly have a certain amount of individual nature of their own, over and above their common characteristics, properties, etc. We have therefore to find out what allowance to make for this (so that we shall at least not act on positively wrong or misplaced expectations), and how we can most quickly discover anything that may seriously matter to us about their individual traits. (iii) It is these specific objects, etc., which are the instruments through which fact-control is exercised on us, even as regards our general expectations and beliefs ; each falsification experienced is itself a singular historical event, happening to us in the form of an individual expectation traversed and overridden by an individual experience-sequence. (iv) In any case we find that large parts of the order of *events* are not capable of being sorted out into the same tidy sets of classes of similar instances as our world of *objects*. Not only is comparison much more difficult in any case, but many kinds of happening have not the same clear boundaries and tend to flow out of one another and into one another in time, in something like a continuum. Others again pass into one another in space, and also in quality, in ways which baffle our pigeon-holing capacity. (v) Furthermore, as we have seen, there are the two comprehensive time-continua, each of them a single and so individual whole, in which we more and more find we have to place everything that happens *to* us and everything that happens *for* us : the personal history of each of us, and the history of our world as a whole. The former we come to see as a part of the latter which is continually intersecting with other parts. But at the same time it is also for each of us central and unique, and its very intersections and interactions with the world and the world-history outside it (through which these chiefly, if not solely, become known to us) are all individual and singular occurrences in our own history. It is equally true indeed that these occurrences mostly recur in regular classes such that they enable us to learn to know the contents of our world (the various kinds of objects and entities in it), and that just because they are so repeatable and recoverable, they become largely merged into the stable and cumulative knowledge they lead to.[1] Nevertheless our every intersection and interaction with our world remains in one aspect a unique dated event in our singular personal story. And we are left with this as one individual whole, and world-history as another individual whole, both of which can only be grasped by us, in their past, present and future dimensions, by unique individual learning and knowledge. That knowledge again is extremely important and valuable to us, and we come to seek each type of it by the methods which we find to be appropriate to it.

(10) From all the foregoing there issues eventually a double causal concern over most of the more significant experiences which confront us, but above all, about those types of *historical happening* which we cannot easily circumscribe within a regular recurrent class, or attach to definite orders of objects, and which tend to implicate, or to draw in with them, the surrounding time-continuum or historical context. We need all the knowledge we can accumulate and bring to bear about the *kind* of any such experience, including above all what controls it and what it controls. But it is also of far-reaching moment to us to be as nearly as possible prepared for *any specific instance* as and when it is going to happen in the context of our own history—which means in most cases, when the correlative occurrence is going to happen in the context of objective history. We want to have seen this instance coming, and to be ready for what it is going to lead to. That holds particularly, of course, for any events that appear likely to impinge in direct form on our own history, but we learn also in increasing degree that there are few large happenings in world-history, above all contemporary and more or less contiguous, which are not apt to have a bearing on our own. And there are few even among the more remote major occurrences in space and time, which have not some light to throw on the course of events that directly impinges on us, and therefore some con-

---

[1] It might be said that there is only one cross-sectional or spatial world of which every object is a part, just as there is only one world-history. But this *cross-sectional* unity is only that of a loose envelope within which we can freely move to and fro, and every object is to a very large extent similar to and interchangeable with a whole " class " of others. World-history, on the other hand, is a single irreversible fabric, in which every happening is knitted (sometimes more, sometimes less closely) to preceding, succeeding and adjacent ones.

E*

tribution to make to our insight into this and foresight relative to it.

Hence our double causal interest and our two distinct forms of causal inquiry, both capable of being applied to every sort of happening, but each tending to be used preferentially for its own appropriate class of occurrence (though with a close inter-relationship and a large overlap). On the one hand we want to know what causes events of *class A* to happen, and what further events they tend to bring with them. On the other hand we wish to learn what has caused the *specific event A^1* to happen here and now, or at a particular time and place (either in my own personal history or in the objective historical context, according to the character of the case). The first can be described as the functional-structural type of causal question, and our corpus of answers, with all accompanying qualifications and complications, makes up a large part of the substance of most of our sciences. The second constitutes the historical type of casual question and clearly finds its outstanding field of application in personal and collective human history, but also provides the main subject-matter for what are often called the historical sciences : geology, evolutionary biology, part of astronomy.

It is plain that the historical sciences, including that of human history, must draw freely on the functional-structural ones, and are in the main dependent on these. But they also have their own further and even more complex and difficult tasks. They cannot be content with general relations ; they must fill in a specific individual pattern, in which all the general relations involved are correctly linked up with one another in time and space, and correctly proportioned to each other, so that in the end any specific event which has to be understood (in the sense of *historical causal* understanding) can be *seen* to flow out of *that* combination of factors, agencies, conditions and actual previous happenings in *that* order and interrelation, at just the time and place at which we find that it *has* happened.

We may note that psychology, although in one aspect a functional-structural science seeking systematic causal knowledge about a *class* of objects, and not about a single history, is obliged to become to a very large extent a historical science, because of the distinctive nature of the class of entities it seeks to know. Its objects are not those physical or physiological organisms, human bodies ; they are human *persons* and their psychic life, which turns out to be in each case a singular cumulative history. These histories have a vast deal in common and thus a *science* of psychology is possible ; but because its units are historical, a causal approach to any happening in them has to pass, at least typically, through their whole story. The fabric of causal explanation or understanding must once more be in terms of a complex of inter-acting agencies, factors and happenings taken in their right order and interrelation, in such wise that their intersection-pattern at any time can be *seen* to lead to whatever actually happens next at that time.

We know how this approach is utilised by the most consciously historical branch of psychology, psycho-analysis, for the fullest insight into the causation of specific happenings at specific times in specific personal life-histories. In so far as it seeks to do this therapeutically, psycho-analysis obviously goes beyond normal theoretical scientific *inquiry* and becomes an applied science. Even so, it uses general relations, like other sciences, but these are themselves of a historical type, and part of a generalised historical pattern. Other branches of psychology, in which practical appli-cation is quite distinct from theoretical inquiry, are obviously not concerned with the individual antecedents of a particular hap-pening at a given time in a particular person, but must no less aim at a cumulative historical account of their subject-matter, even if in a much more general form. Psychology as a whole can in the last resort only be the study of typical human life-histories in different settings, together with their typical deviations from one another both in similar and in different settings, and the correla-tion of these deviations both with differences of endowment, or inherited psychic constitution, and with differences in setting. And the basic pattern must throughout be that of *cumulative historical interaction* between the individual subject and his setting. (We have here considered only the more advanced weft of human *cognitive* history in our own society, under relatively favourable conditions which allow a reasonable degree of individual catching-up with its more developed cognitive levels. The main historical failures to achieve this pattern, or deviations from it, and their causes and conditions, together with their survivals in our society, can easily be fitted into our story and have been adumbrated at various points ; but space does not allow for a detailed account.)

(11) The foregoing does not pretend to be more than the roughest and most incomplete sketch of the immense theme of all the experiential material which enters into and makes up our causal sense. It should however suffice to indicate the lines along which the sketch could readily be carried very much further, and

at the same time to establish our essential point : that as in the case of the existence of objects and of the objective world, so in that of the reality of causal relations as common sense believes in it, there is a vast body of convergent, cumulative experience, learning from such experience, and incessant testing and confirmation of that learning, which accounts for every aspect and component of our belief and unshakeably sustains it. (Incidentally the whole of our technological civilisation, in which every day a myriad *causal operations* of the most diverse kinds are carried out under controlled conditions with automatic success, provides its own eloquent daily witness to the same effect.) And of course, as we have already emphasised, the entire structure of our causal knowledge stands as a further development, and a further confirmation, of our belief in the objective world on which it is all built ; so that this in turn takes over, in addition to all its other supports, the full massiveness and solidity and strength of that vast structure of cumulative experience and cumulatively verified truths.

However, we must conclude by recognising again that, as distinct from the great systematic body of our scientific causal knowledge, our everyday notion of causality as such has remained in a state of lamentable muddle. Everything that is necessary is there, and *can* emerge when occasion arises, but certain overriding confusions and errors are apt to keep far short of adequacy what in fact emerges on most ordinary occasions. Our assumption that there is such a thing as " the " (single) cause of a given effect is always misguiding us into fastening on some particular element in the total causal-and-conditioning pattern, and neglecting the rest. The only ways in which we testify to the full truth which is in us is by frequently picking on different fragments on different occasions, and also—yet more paradoxically—by selecting different fragments from one another on the same occasion, and quarrelling with one another as to which is " the " true cause. To understand fully what is happening, and why, we must indeed acknowledge that the element which is chosen in a particular case will usually tend to be that which happens to be the most relevant to the angle from which we are approaching the case, the type of interest we are bringing to it, etc. But this cannot alter the fact that the pictures which thus emerge are generally more or less badly distorted, just because we believe them to be sufficient or complete. We may pick out as " the " cause virtually any factor which enters into a causal situation or can in any circumstances become relevant to it : the initiating event, the operative substance or agency, the character of the substance or medium acted upon, the presence of any one of the predisposing or even the permissive conditions, even the absence of some particular preventive cause, or for that matter anything which, *if* it had happened to be different, would have made the outcome different. In such cases of complex causation as the larger events of human history, World War I or II, the French Revolution, the Reformation, etc., we are specially apt to run riot in the diversity of the types of causal factor which we advocate as " the " cause. But there the excess of ill tends to provide its own remedy, and most latter-day historians are perfectly clear that an adequate account of the way in which any one of these vast and complex happenings came about, *and pursued its actual course* (the questions are inseparable), must bring in and properly marshal an immense *concourse* of factors, conditions and events that made their contribution on different scales and at different levels and within different space and time horizons towards the total situation and made it *flow* into the shape it did. In other words, cumulative systematic attention to a concrete case does eventually bring out, and assemble together, most if not all the components of our complete causal sense.

However, there are many other confusions which beset our everyday causal notions besides those arising from the fallacy of " the " cause. No detailed study of all of them is possible here, but we may particularly note the way in which the combination of vagueness with muddle leads to the application of the causal question-form in all sorts of situations in which it practically loses its meaning. This form is in fact apt to be used about virtually anything : someone may ask about " the cause " of a property, or a quality, or a location, or a relation, or an aspect, or even an object or substance or for that matter the whole world. It is often very difficult to say what is meant by such a question, i.e. what the questioner really wants to know. Sometimes a near approach to a genuine causal inquiry can be secured by trying the substitution of the notion of " determining " : what (in the way of structure, composition, etc.) determines the presence of this particular property, quality, or whatever it may be ? This of course is the converse of the notion of causal dependence, and is, as we have seen, closely allied to the authentic idea of active causality, to which it is indeed the static complement. But if it is not carefully and clearly defined, it may likewise lose itself all-too-readily in vagueness. In effect, at times it is not possible to achieve sense even with the help of that substitution, and the question as put may be regarded as hardly more than one of those automatic extensions of a habit by analogy which are bound sooner or later to carry it beyond the bounds not only of validity but of significance.

What concerns us more closely, however, than this fading out is a specific confusion which is almost ubiquitous. It arises in fact very plausibly from the actual overlap of the notion of causality with that of explanation—an overlap which frequently leads us not merely to confuse but to fuse the two. But though there is this overlap, the notion of explanation has its own very distinctive meaning, and its own fundamental role in the whole of our cognitive development. An endeavour to bring out its proper psychological background and significance both as related to and as fully distinguishable from that of causality will occupy us in the next chapter.

CHAPTER VII

THE PSYCHOLOGY OF PUZZLEMENT AND OF EXPLANATION

(1) We are to a large extent taking up again in this chapter the thread of Chapter III, which dealt with the experiential basis for our distinction between truth and falsity and the main processes by which we build up and test our knowledge. The notion of explanation plays an extremely important part in the more developed phases of these processes, but that part is apt to be either missed altogether, or at best very inadequately understood, owing to the current confusions between causal inquiry or information and explanation. More generally the latter concept is probably the least discussed and considered of our fundamental epistemological ideas, partly again because it is too readily assumed that discussions of causality cover all the relevant ground. Its own very special import tends thus to be completely overlooked. What we shall suggest is that in its distinctive sense, the notion of explanation completes in a most essential respect the story, sketched in outline in Chapter III, of *how* we learn from our experience, in contrast to Chapters IV to VI, which were concerned with the two outstanding aspects of *what* we learn from our experience. An adequate approach to explanation will be found to bring its own contribution in support of our general thesis.

(2) The first task, however, is to get both the distinction and the chief ground for the confusion between the ideas of explanation and of causality fully clear.

The latter concept (together with the cognate one of dependence) is, as we have seen, fundamentally that of a *relation between objective facts*, or if we prefer, of *a characteristic of the objective world* (that events arise out of others and give rise to further ones ; that agencies introduced or applied in specific fields start characteristic changes in those fields ; that the continuance of a certain feature of a state of affairs is bound up with the presence and continuance of certain other features, etc.).

On the other hand the notion of explanation is that of a *particular type of knowledge or information*, or rather of knowledge with a *particular function*, relative to a previous cognitive situation into which it is newly introduced. Causal information very often and very powerfully exercises this " explanatory " function ; but it is far from the only kind of information that does so. And furthermore, the role it assumes when it serves as explanation is quite different, as we shall see, from that which characterises it as the answer to straightforward causal questions. The important fact about an explanation, whatever the nature of the information it consists of, is its functional relation to a previous cognitive state.

(3) This state is that of puzzlement, or nonplusment. Nothing is commoner or more familiar, from early childhood throughout the years up to the most advanced levels of human knowledge, social as well as individual. Its obvious first root is, once again, the experience of falsified expectation, and the state immediately following on this. But it does not assume its more specific forms until a certain degree of organisation and consolidation of our experience has been reached and until the child is able and ready to focus some measure of continued attention on his falsified expectations—or, what is by then almost the same thing, his confrontations with very *unexpected* findings or happenings in contexts with which he is generally familiar.

There is, however, evidence of the characteristic state of cognitive puzzlement by the third year, and by the fourth it has usually found its way to typical explicit expression in the child's " why " questions—or, more accurately, in a certain class of these. By this type of question he is essentially voicing his perplexity over a sudden clash between his previous settled beliefs or assumptions and some present finding, and seeking an answer which will somehow remove or overcome that sense of clash. An " explanation " is primarily *new or additional information of a kind which will relieve puzzlement and resolve any (real or apparent) cognitive clash.*

(4) We cannot be too careful here not to be misled by the various distinct meanings of the term " why " and still more by our chronic failure to keep them properly apart. We tend to regard the term as particularly denoting the causal question-form ; but in a pre-scientific guise, with an archaic bias towards teleological assumptions, that is, with an implicit belief that for everything there is in the background an answer or " explanation " in terms of purpose, design or at least " reason." This has led to the formula so much favoured by many scientists that science is not concerned with the (pre-scientific) question " why," but only with the question " how."

In fact it is evident that one meaning of the word " why " is definitely that of inquiry about motives or purposes. This of course is perfectly appropriate for *human actions* and equally so for very many *products of human activities*. Furthermore it must plainly represent the first meaning of the word which the child picks up ; adults do not talk to him about their states of cognitive perplexity, but they do need to find out from him (where it is not self-evident) " why " he is crying, or " why " he is doing or not doing this or that. The whole context of the question usually conveys to him what is wanted of him, and very often he is only waiting to express his trouble himself, so that it is very natural that after a time he gets the full purport of that introductory sound. He is no doubt also helped towards this by constantly hearing it used in the same way by the adults round him, speaking to one another and receiving characteristic answers. And so eventually he begins to use the word himself, for the same purpose and in the same fashion. He thereupon finds in fact that it is a wonderful open sesame. The comings and goings and actions of his mother and the rest of his family are both the most important things in his early life and also, outside certain established routines, the most variable and unpredictable, as regards both their antecedents and their outcomes. From his own unaided experiences of them it is extremely difficult for him to know either when to expect them or what to expect of them. But " why " provides him with a key which helps him in both these ways.

It is equally natural that thereafter he should seek to work this key for all it is worth. The first obvious extension is from the purposes of action to the purposes of objects, which are so often bound up with human activities or seen being shaped or produced by them. And inevitably the child does not know where to draw the line, or indeed that there is a line to be drawn. He can only come to know this by gradual learning. He applies his " why " automatically to every successive thing which arouses his interest, with the expectation that he will get a similar illuminating-feeling answer. And very often, indeed, he obtains it even where he should not. In any event purpose shades readily into function, so that although the child slowly begins to discover that there are a good many kinds of situation where he cannot secure the type of answer which he was expecting, the sorting out tends to remain for some time—if not always—imperfect and incomplete.

(5) We are not here concerned with the complete natural history of this process ; what we must note particularly, however, is that in spite of the very powerful start which this meaning of

" why " secures and the wide domain in which it maintains its full significance and validity, a quite distinct second meaning usually breaks through to the consciousness of the child as early as the second half of the fourth year, or at any rate during the fifth year. He might indeed find opportunities in the longer run of gradually picking it up from the talk of adults with one another, but a far more important factor is that there is something in him seeking to be expressed, and various easy transitions readily lead him from the uses of " why " to which he is already accustomed to this further one which directly relates itself to the waiting need.

The transition emerges immediately from one central element in the very situations which start off his " why's " of inquiry for motive or purpose. As we have noted, he is led to ask them about activities to which he is not accustomed, for which he is not prepared, which suddenly or newly invade his field of attention. And of course all the more about any which seem *contrary* to what he usually expects, or was at the moment expecting. Answers which enable him to see where such unexpected or anti-expected activities have come from and are going to, and so to prepare himself for them for the future, and still more, answers which reconcile him even to anti-expected ones by showing that, in spite of their anti-expectedness, they are going to work out all right for him, can bring him not only a sense of illumination and understanding, but also a considerable feeling of relief. Anything new and unfamiliar is liable to arouse anxiety, and anything directly *contrary* to expectation and preparation tends automatically to do so.[1] Hence the relief due to replies which usually fit what is happening into the general pattern of familiar security of the child, and quite often show it to lead to some new positive satisfaction for him.

These answers will, moreover, often call his attention to new facts or features of the total situation, of which he was not aware, and which may provide a clear bridge between his previous expectation and what is actually being done contrary to this. That lesson, too, is not lost on the child, harmonising as it does with many similar discoveries of his own, of the kind we have already described.

From this aspect of his " why's " about the motives and purposes of actions, i.e., the initiating element of unexpectedness or anti-

---

[1] A joke or any unexpected comical turn of events is once more the exception which proves the rule. The element of tension which often precedes laughter, and the corresponding element of relief in the laughter, have frequently been noted.

expectedness in them, it is only a short step to the use of the " why " question as a means of seeking similar relief and help in any other experience of unexpectedness or anti-expectedness, irrespective of its source. The stress now falls on the clash and at-a-lossness as such, and the demand is for a bridge or key which will allow the child to make the clashing or disconcerting experience fit in.

And we actually find that from about the turn of the fourth year, intelligent children ask " why " questions which clearly have nothing to do with human actions and their motives, purposes or other causes, but express directly the child's perplexity in the presence of a divergence, or apparent divergence, from what he has come to regard as the established properties or behaviour or pattern of things. The more firmly such a pattern has become rooted and the more strongly it is organised, the greater is his perplexity and the clearer the purport of his appeal for adult help. From an earlier comprehensive study of children's " why " questions[1] I may quote just two illustrative instances. A boy aged 4 ; 1 asks " Why doesn't the ink run out when you hold up a fountain pen ? " And " Why don't we see two things with our two eyes ? " The interested reader may be referred to this study for many other examples and for a detailed analysis of a number of them. What I have called the epistemic meaning of " why " is there fully discussed and I believe established.

(6) We need merely glance here at two further points which are more fully developed in that study.

(i) We have only so far considered two major meanings of the term " why ", but there are various others which branch out from the same root, but later become badly tangled up with one another. We are not concerned with most of them here, except as sources of confusion. (*a*) From " why " as inquiry about the causes (motives or purposes) of human actions, there is a ready passage to the use of " why " equally for the causes of other happenings. As we have already noted, this tends to carry with it, especially at the beginning, the automatic assumption that these other causes will also be of the nature of motives or purposes, but whilst that assumption is largely shed later on (at any rate in all the contexts where it is quite obviously inappropriate), the use of the *term* " why " for every sort of causal question is still retained. The situation is further complicated by the fact that even human

---

[1] Published as an appendix to Susan Isaacs' *Intellectual Growth in Young Children* (Routledge 1930).

actions are often found to have causes which cannot be thought of as motives or purposes. And also, as we have seen, by the fact that the concept of purpose becomes separated from that of human action as such and extended, in one direction, to the *products* of human activities, and in another to all living or organic entities and their make-up and behaviour, with a partial and gradual transition to the wider notion of function.[1] (*b*) From " why " as inquiry about the motives of human active behaviour, there is yet another line of development leading to the more specialised use of the term, first for the *motives* or *purposes* of particular pieces of speech-behaviour ("Why do you say this ? " = " What makes you say this ? "), and then for the *justifications* or *reasons* or grounds (as it were " logical " motives or causes) of particular statements. This last development links up again to some extent with the aspect of unexpectedness or anti-expectedness in the first " why's " about behaviour : the challenge for " logical " or supporting and justifying motives arises first and foremost when a statement is unexpected or anti-expected and therefore difficult to accept or to fit in with the hearer's knowledge, or believed knowledge. He therefore asks, at any rate to begin with, for some bridge or key to show how it *can be* fitted in. (*c*) There are also diverse uses of " why " of a merely affective or exclamatory type : sheer surprise, vexation, protest, etc., pointing back plainly enough, once more, to the original situations of disconcerting unexpectedness or anti-expectedness from which the word takes its rise.

(ii) Partly overlapping with the previous point, we may note an important general distinction between the various types of question asked by the child—a distinction which will lead us straight on to the further deployment of the concept of explanation. Once more there is confusion, as well as distinction, and the confusion arises chiefly from the ambiguities of " why " and the fact that " why " questions (of different kinds) fall on both sides of the division.

In effect we can draw a clear contrast of *type* between questions of every sort, including most classes of " why's ", which seek *predefined information* of a particular order, and the one great outstanding group of " why's " that seeks that peculiar unpredefinable category of information—information about which we

---

[1] The confusion between cause-seeking and explanation-seeking "why's " is made still worse by the further fact that some kinds of cause, particularly intervening or preventing ones, provide one of the commonest types of explanatory information. But this factor will be more fully considered below.

only know in advance the psychological function it is intended to serve—which we call explanation.

The former type of question develops when some of the first large lines of organisation of our experience have already been laid down ; and it serves as an extremely fruitful and powerful means of consolidating and expanding each such realm of incipient knowledge. The child picks up one by one a series of separate question-forms, each standing for a distinctive order of information applicable over a wide area of experience, and learns to use each of them as an instrument for gathering information of that order about one after another of a great variety of experience-foci. He thus knows in advance the *kind* of answer he wants, and his very question reflects and expresses this knowledge. Thus each such question-form becomes a key to a particular growing body of information (obviously both inviting and facilitating regular comparison and orderly, systematic arrangement).

The first to emerge (and therefore the least clear), is of course the familiar " What is . . . (that) ? " This signifies minimally : " What is it called ? " But the background interest is usually : " What manner of thing is it ? " To what class does it belong ? —At the beginning, naturally, quite new classes have constantly to be supplied. This is most often done by just providing a new name ; that then serves as the nucleus of a new group, to which further members (within the appropriate range of variation) are added by re-application of the now familiar name-word.[1]

Later and better-defined question-forms of the same order are : What makes . . . ? — Of what is . . . made ? — Where . . . ? — Where from . . . ? Who . . . ? How . . . ? When . . . ? How large . . . ? How many . . . ? etc., etc. And also : " Why ? " in any one of its several straightforward information-seeking senses. All these are ways of *adding* to a particular class of information the child already possesses, and at the same time of filling in a particular type of gap. The use of each form testifies to the child's awareness of that specific gap in what he knows about some subject-matter he is interested in ; he is clear about what he wants to find out to complete his picture in that respect, and asks for it. He may carry some of the question-forms rather beyond their significant bounds (and has to learn these from such trial and error), but he does not usually use any of them where it is entirely out of place. They are prepared headings to be filled

---

[1] We are all amused at times by some of the odd uses which children make of our cues ; but we less often stop to understand the exact logic behind the process.

in on suitable occasions and constitute both one part of the desirable knowledge to be procured about specific things, and one class of knowledge to be procured about many things. The discovery and mastery of these question-forms provides the child with a very rapid and easy means of multiplying his information— or at any rate, in his early days, as he flits from use to use, of multiplying his sense of information—and though his first eager interest in some of them may flag, they become a permanent acquisition as an expression of the consciousness of a particular kind of ignorance (where it is significant), and so the first step towards the search for the appropriate knowledge.

Between all these types of question and the *explanation*-seeking " why," we can establish, at least in principle, a very plain and marked distinction. The latter emerges later and has quite a different background, function and aim. The child is *not* asking for a predefined type of information, because the whole crux of his state is that he does not know what sort of information he wants. He is at a loss : the previous organisation of his thought, instead of carrying him on (as in all the above cases), has suddenly let him down. There is a clash or contradiction between what he now finds, or seems to find, and what he had previously been brought to believe, and he does not know what to do about it. He cannot straight away give up or modify his previous belief or scheme of beliefs ; all the past successes which have consolidated it into what it now is speak against that. Yet he has somehow to deal with the irresistible fact of the present experience which clashes. His " why " question is, as we have said, an appeal for a bridge or a key : for some X of new information, he has no idea of what kind, which, when he gets it, will enable him to extricate himself from his present deadlock.

This is the primary burden of meaning of the " why " of puzzlement and appeal for an explanation. Something of that state of mind always survives, but at the same time there is also an inevitable development which goes some way to blur again, in our everyday practice, the sharp antithesis of principle between predefined information-seeking and our quest for some explanatory X. What supervenes is of course our cumulative experience of actual explanations received, and the consequent progressive sorting out of these into different types. Thus we get a number of secondary groups of information-seeking questions, and in particular the class we have already referred to, the pursuit of special kinds of causal information which have often been found to have the needed explanatory value—most obviously the search for unsuspected intervening causes, which may perfectly " explain " why something expected did not happen, or something unexpected did. The " why " form has very naturally remained strongly attached to this type of quest, since it is used for causes anyhow, and possesses a special aptness for the case of unsuspected or unexpected causes.

Apart, however, from this specific order of derivative information-seeking, even the " why's " of authentic puzzlement tend after a time not to remain completely indeterminate, but only indeterminate as between the various previously experienced types of explanation. Nevertheless this is no more than a tendency. The puzzlement is there, and though we can set out a number of alternative ways in which it may be resolvable, with a high probability that it will in fact be resolved in one of these ways, our actual state when what we are seeking is an *explanation* remains one of uncertain questioning. Till we have found it (and verified it !), we just cannot prejudge what, and of what kind, the " explanation " will be. And indeed, even apart from unknown possibilities (which we cannot in advance rule out), the known types of alternatives are so different and disparate that until one of them stands out as the probable answer, our general familiarity with them can do little if anything to relieve our perplexed state. To some of these disparate alternatives we must now briefly turn.

(7) We have already emphasised that an explanation is essentially new and mediating information which will somehow remove the clash or gap, real or apparent, between a present experience, or apparent present experience, and pre-existing beliefs. We have indicated in our earlier account of falsified expectations that the situation may be resolved in the simplest possible way by the discovery (whether supplied by anyone else or made by oneself) that one had misinterpreted one's present experience—that is, misperceived, or misjudged what one was perceiving, but as soon as this was corrected, the whole difficulty and apparent clash disappeared. We have also pointed out that, at the other extreme, our new discordant experience may obstinately stay put, and we may find that nothing else will serve but a sharp correction, or even sometimes a far-reaching reconstruction, of our present scheme of beliefs. In such cases it is usually also of importance to us to establish how we went wrong. But the answer may of course just be that on our previous data we could not tell any better. Our accepted belief might even have been a brilliantly successful

theory which had long seemed to deal with every relevant case we could think of (like the Newtonian system). And yet it might finally come up against findings which refused to fit in and which at length suggested some radically different theory or belief-scheme that was in equal accord with the previous data, but *also* fully explained the new facts, i.e. made it possible to deduce (and so to predict or anticipate) these—and led to the prediction and verification of many more besides.

Between these two opposite extremes, we may get any one or more of quite a large number of intermediate types of resolution. We may learn from others or find for ourselves all kinds of factors which we had not taken into account : unconsidered qualifying circumstances or intervening causes ; missing links, either in the form of facts or in that of rules ; an unrecognised but bridging class-subsumption ; distinguishing or delimiting features, etc. And finally, we may be left with our perplexity and problem on our hands, and may recognise this, but may also fall victims to some formula that means little more, but may get put forward as if it were itself an " explanation " : chance, or the original natures or irreducible differences of things. A closer examination of each of these alternative possibilities, and indeed a full and systematic study of the whole field, would be repaying but cannot be attempted here.

These are all legitimate outcomes of our states of perplexity. But besides these, we have to recognise the existence of a great host of what must definitely be regarded as pseudo-explanations. Some of these are aberrations of language, particularly philosophic ; others are old-established myths, usually fed from early affective sources, and in some cases surrounded and defended by an immense cloud-screen of philosophic-linguistic pseudo-explanations.[1] The latter include all explanations by " ideas " and their " implications," verbal paraphrases, reified abstractions, faculties, etc., and much that appears more subtle and sophisticated but is not at bottom very different. Detailed consideration of these aberrant forms is again beyond our scope here. What is relevant for us is only the contrast between explanations which

[1] This comment does not of course imply any *a priori* rejection of religious philosophies or cosmologies which are prepared to subject themselves to the same standards of evidence and the same tests as " scientific " explanatory theories : i.e. that are prepared like these to submit themselves to real evidence and real tests outside themselves. Unless indeed they claim to be based on sources of knowledge which are quite independent of any experiential evidence or tests ; in which case the sources themselves have to be validated by some sort of independent or objective test. See further below and Chapter VIII.

explain, and those others so called which do not begin to be able to do so. That is to say, the contrast between explanations which (a) are true and can be verified to be true, and (b) at the same time fulfil the explanatory function they are intended to fulfil (i.e. perform the particular piece of integration which our initial perplexity or problem called for), and all those pretended ones which fail to comply with one or both of these conditions, and thus either do not qualify even as potential explanations or completely fail to make good as actual ones. And what is of vital importance for our whole approach here is precisely the adequacy or otherwise of our *standard* of explanation, as the key either to the premature silting up and closure of the progress of our learning, or to its unlimited cumulative advance.

All the foregoing applies equally to the cognitive development of the individual and that of the race. But if an entire community has become enclosed in some narrow circle of limited information and limiting pseudo-explanation, individuals stand little chance of breaking through this. On the other hand even if a society as a whole has found its way to the open growth of knowledge, it is still possible for individuals to lose theirs, or to be led astray, or to suffer one or another form of early arrest of growth.

(8) The epistemic why-question marks the parting of the ways. Any experience for which there is no place in our pre-existing scheme of beliefs or world-picture, whether general or local, is a challenge to us. The child addresses his " why " to parent or teacher or friendly adult, because they already know so much more and may be able to deal with this challenge, whether by correcting any element of error or by telling him something new which serves as a bridge. The adult may have to seek his own answer or explanation where he can, and if he is an investigating scientist working on the present social boundaries of knowledge, he can only address the question to himself.

But the point now is what happens next. The state of challenge or questioning is one of unrest, of uneasiness, of alert seeking ; if something is found which is *accepted* as the explanation, the uneasiness is allayed, the alertness subsides, the mind returns to a state of rest. Thus the inquirer's *criteria of what constitutes a valid explanation* will determine in what circumstances he will settle down, in what others he will go on with his search. The child is of course chiefly dependent in this matter on his parents and teachers ; he can hardly do other than to take over their *criteria* of explanation together with their actual explanations ; it is from the latter that he will mainly fashion the former. The investigating scientist, on the other hand, will have absorbed, in the course of his training, the criteria implicit in the method and tradition of his science. The ordinary person's we know to be largely inarticulate, incomplete and imperfect. The scientist's we have every reason for thinking substantially sound, since the whole history of science is the history of learning processes which have found their way to uninhibited expansion, systematic self-correction and cumulative growth. But even the scientist's criteria are not often explicit and fully worked out ; indeed, if he is asked to say what he means by an explanation, or when and how an explanation explains, he may at best start with a conventional formula, but quite possibly he will do little better than to fumble and grope ; and either way it will not be long before he finds himself involved in every sort of philosophic difficulty.

The whole *theory of scientific theories* is in fact still in a parlous state, and many of the formulae repeated by one scientist after another, if he has to pronounce on this awkward quasi-philosophic topic, represent untenable crudities dating back to certain early attempts to rescue science at all costs, even that of elementary sense, from the entanglements of philosophy.[1] The state of professional philosophic debate on the same subject is however no better, and here there is not even at work any safeguarding *functional* criterion of valid explanation, any more than that precondition of progressive discussion, a stable and effective theory of truth. Our suggestion has been from the start that an adequate *psychological* account of truth and falsity is the first foundation on which all our approach to knowledge and its problems must be built. This is brought out once more with particular force by the contemporary position in regard to the concept of explanation. It is often stated and almost always assumed that an explanation must be true because it explains this or that. The fact is of course that an explanation can only explain anything *if* it is true. Its ability to " explain " some set of facts may, if adequate criteria of what this means have been applied and the offered suggestion

---

[1] A favourite formula, of a fantastic degree of inadequacy, is that of scientific theories and concepts as more or less arbitrary inventions intended to " order " our experience, and competing with one another only according to the degree of " success " with which they " order " a maximum span of experience with a minimum of conceptual or theoretical apparatus. This no doubt removes any philosophically troublesome reference to *truth* from our scientific theories. But it completely disregards every ascertainable fact about the origin, history, functioning and mode of test of every actual scientific notion and hypothesis.

or hypothesis fulfils the minimum conditions of potential truth,[1] establish some *presumption* of its probable truth. But until there has either been direct verification of the suggested " explanation," or the assemblage of a very strong body of varied *independent* findings all of which it, *and no other hypothesis that can be thought of*, will explain, one cannot go beyond saying that *if* it were true, it *would* explain the given set of facts.

The temporal-correspondence account of truth and falsity set out here, buttressed by our general description of our learning processes and of the main burden of what we have learnt by these, leads to a clear and objective basis both for our notion of explanation and for its functional history and operative criteria, in the closest accordance with the most searching and fruitful scientific *practice*. The way in which our account of the place and development of explanation in our cognitive growth takes up the story of truth and falsity and of our learning processes in general, and carries it further to the level of our fullest scientific achievement, is yet another confirmation of the validity of our approach.

---

[1] It will be clear that the basic minimum condition of potential truth of any proposition, on our view, is that it must be *capable* of being confronted, point by point, in the shape of a set of clearly and unequivocally formulated anticipations, with a controlling objective context, i.e. a context of appropriate primary experience, which must either verify or falsify these anticipations. Single deducible expectations do not suffice : they might be deducible from a host of other propositions, or their background may be wholly vague. *Every part* of the content of the " explanation " must be translatable into such expectations—just as is every part of the content of our belief in objects and an objective world, or every part of the content of every authentic scientific theory.

CHAPTER VIII

THE BEARINGS OF AN ADEQUATE PSYCHOLOGY OF KNOWLEDGE ON THE PHILOSOPHIC THEORY OF KNOWLEDGE

(1) We have underlined from the start that an adequate empirical account of the psychological facts of knowledge must come before any philosophic consideration or evaluation of the problems of knowledge. Assuming now that we have brought out, at least in the broadest way, the central psychological facts of our learning history—*how* we learn, and *what* in the main we have learnt, about our experience-world—what place is left for the philosophic theory of knowledge ? How should its problems now be formulated and approached ?

(2) Before, however, we can give any sort of answer to this question, we shall do well to repair, however briefly, certain omissions in our factual account (only just touched upon earlier) ; certain facts, possibilities and questions which are still obviously matters for specific empirical inquiry, within the framework of a proper empirical psychology of knowledge, and so again should precede our philosophic approach, as part of the *material* for it, instead of being left over as its exclusive preserve.

But to make sure of getting our proportions right, let us first pass in review again the solid and massive structure of what we have already established. We have so far concentrated on certain basic learning processes, the foundational knowledge they provide, and everything that can be, and thereafter is, cumulatively built on them. We have seen that we (individually and collectively) learn primarily from undergoing various kinds of experiences in various constellations, groupings and relations ; from retaining, after similar recurrences, the patterns of many of these ; from reviving, upon the recurrence of a similar experience-segment, the whole of some pattern, and projecting the rest ahead of us as what we expect now to experience or to be able to experience ; and from then actually getting, for the most part, the expected pattern, but often also suffering the further all too distinctive experience not only of a more or less different one, but also, of the shock or jar of its clash with our expectation. This forces the latter into the open, in one and the same breath, as *merely* our belief, and a *wrong* belief, whilst the frequent occurrence of that kind of pulling-up starts us off and guides us towards endless closer distinctions within our experience and more watchful limitation of our beliefs. Thus we are forced concurrently to *expand*, to *articulate*, and to *revise* the patterns of our expectations and beliefs in order to meet more and more adequately and dependably the cumulatively expanding patterns of our actual experience. These processes go on the whole time from the earliest infancy of each of us, in the most varied forms and combinations, and from at least the second year onwards, are compounded with the accumulated social heritage of learning of our whole society, built up in the same way. Every aspect of them contributes to elaborate in us a great central scheme of expectations and assumptions which we later call that of belief in an external world governed by causality. That is, a world of continuing objects and objective happenings of which we are object-members ourselves and which controls our experiences of every kind, but most directly and distinctively those of the perceptual type ; and a world of which every component is found to be bound up with every other in relations of mutual dependence, control and interaction, within a single comprehensive history.

This central pattern of expectations and beliefs is particularly reinforced by all our local experiences of error and " mere " false belief, which in fact support its main tenor. Accordingly it forms the foundation on which our future learning attitude itself is built : it is more and more borne in upon us that for *reliable* and *sufficient* knowledge we must go out and subject ourselves to the further control of that world ; we must go on and on exploring and investigating it, in order to extend the content and range of our picture of it and to fill in more and more fully the network of its internal connections and relations. That is how in effect we proceed to build up the vast bodies of dependable knowledge which (in virtue of this character) we call our sciences. Their great principle of growth is that of voluntarily accepted and sought *fact-control*, both in the form of fact-exploration and in that of fact-test. Their chief underlying assumption is that if we are to have both *true* beliefs and an adequate volume of them, we can never sufficiently press on with our inquiries into the relevant fields of fact, or carefully enough test our beliefs and *seek out* any latent errors in them. And even when we have done all we can think of in this way, we must still be ready to assume that there may be at least elements of error left in them, or some of them might even still be substantially mistaken, and we must be prepared therefore at all times to meet half-way any possible new indications of such error, and to submit ourselves afresh to the most searching further fact-control we can devise in order to bring anything that is still unsound in our beliefs (and that may point the way to further flaws) into the full light of day.

All this can manifestly only rest on the acknowledgment of a world of fact ; meaning, as we have seen, realms of experience which stand for that world and through which—*by suitable attentional activities and the ensuing receptivity*—we can submit ourselves to its control. The control is always through one of the experience-orders we have called primary : in the exploring aspect of our learning activities the stress falls on the collection of further primary experience ; in the testing aspect, on the confrontation of an expectation or representation of a pattern of such experience with whatever actual primary content next comes to us, in order to establish correspondence or non-correspondence (or of course any mixture or combination of the two, or *degree* of non-correspondence).

And whilst we find that the main arena in which we can indefinitely expand our knowledge, or assemblage of true beliefs, is that of our perceptual experience (moving always within the field we call the spatial one and centred on the control-foci we later call objects and objective events, processes, etc.), we can readily establish that we also form true beliefs or knowledge about all our other primary experiences which lack any such controlling foci and thus do not stand for, or in any sense represent " objective " actualities outside themselves. These include first of all our own states of feeling, craving, fearing, etc., which we regard as essentially our own subjective history. We can form anticipation patterns of feeling-constellations, desire sequences, etc.; we can project these ahead of us at given moments of time, in the presence of suitable primary-experience-segments of the same kind, and we can then find either correspondence or non-correspondence with the further primary feeling experiences, cravings, etc., which actually come. Such beliefs, and the regular bodies of information we build up from them, are then distinctively psychological knowledge. We have seen, indeed, that what we call physical knowledge is in one sense psychological too, since it has to be built up through perceptual experience both in the first learning and in the final testing, and it plays its own essential part, too, in our psychological history. It has, however, the *additional* coefficient or attribute of being objective (which we have noted is itself a condensate of a vast number of convergent primary experiences). And when we are concerned with extending and testing this mode of knowledge in its own field, we abstract from its psychological side and focus wholly on its content in that field, whilst on the other hand we tend to think of as peculiarly " psychological " the knowledge of our " merely " subjective states which (however caused) do not directly manifest or stand for anything outside themselves.

(3) That summarises very roughly the central and fundamental learning pattern on which we have focused our attention here. It binds together in a coherent whole our incessant, automatic, cumulative working criterion of truth and falsity, and all the vast body of dependably true beliefs, or genuine knowledge, or science, which we build up round it. It leaves equal room for our physical sciences (essentially perceptual, or if we prefer, perception-controlled) and for psychology, but it may well seem to suggest not only that the former have also their psychological side, but also that *whatever does not belong within their field, can only fall within that of psychology.*

However, we have not claimed that this is the whole story of our knowledge, even though it is obviously a very far-reaching one. It is very clear and very firmly knit, and it covers the characteristic history of our empirical scientific knowledge of the physical world, whilst leaving room for a parallel history of our specific " psychological " knowledge. Moreover it provides us with a sharp working distinction between (i) thought that makes no claim to truth (fantasy) (ii) thought that claims truth, but only within the subjective field (representation or description of " merely " psychological facts or happenings), and (iii) thought that claims truth in the field of objective or physical fact, disclosed to us by the special type of experience we call perceptual. We have seen just what this last claim means, how it operates, how it is tested, and how liable it is to fail under that test. We have also noted that our first type of truth-claim (ii) is of essentially the same nature and subject to the same kind of test, though within a much more restricted domain.

But we are left now with two orders of question. First, have we any sources of thought other than those we have so far considered claiming truth in the same fields of either " merely " psychological or else objective or physical fact ? And how do any such other sources compare with those already noted for scope and reliability? —Secondly, have we any sources of thought claiming truth in some other field, or of some other kind, than we have so far envisaged ? If so, what is that other field or kind, what does the claimed " truth " of a particular thought in relation to it signify, and how is it tested or measured ? And of course both these orders of question, once they are positively answered, lead automatically to this further one : How far are any of these claims *established*—certainly, or probably, or in any degree ? For *all* our experience suggests that it is always possible for truth-claims to be mistaken, and that any thought, unless we can show otherwise, might be either an error or a mere fantasy.

(4) It has already been made plain that these large topics cannot here be pursued in any detail. The main points that concern us are their relations to empirical psychology on the one hand and to philosophic epistemology on the other. We have contended that at least some of them should, like our previous themes, be matters for empirical psychology, at any rate *before* philosophic inquiry is applied to them. It only remains now to suggest that this is true of all of the above questions, those of the second group as much as those of the first. The only difference between them is in effect that the second group calls for some preliminary clarification : the clearer and sharper our picture of truth-claims in the " merely " psychological and the objective (perception-controlled) fields, and of our ways of measuring and testing them, the more ground we have for insisting on an equal clarity and sharpness of outline of such truth-claims as by hypothesis do not refer to either of the above fields, and thus leave the whole issue of what they do refer to on our hands. And the above preliminary work must also, in the first place at least, be a matter for empirical inquiry ; for the very first issue is : what does anyone who makes such claims (verbally) *mean* by them ? We need, to begin with, a *description* or *account* of what the proponents of such claims are thinking or representing or picturing. They are making sounds or using signs ; our starting assumption is that they are not referring to anything in all that large and familiar realm we call the objective or physical world, or even to anything in that more restricted world we call that of human feeling states and other subjective or merely psychological conditions. What precisely then *do* the users of those sounds or signs mean by them ?

If this question can be intelligibly answered, we can then go on to the others, namely how we can assess whether and how far given types of truth-claim in these special realms are valid or justified or dependable. And how any specific claim comes out when so assessed. These again are, in the first place, topics for local psychological inquiry : for we are still and always dealing with phenomena which, whatever else they may be besides, are at least psychological *to begin with* (just like perception itself). In effect they occur in the same single interconnected historical context of our experience or our states as all other psychological phenomena, and must be both distinguished from them and related to them. And that in turn means that, just like these, they must be systematically studied when they occur and as they occur, so that in this their psychological aspect we can build up an adequate fabric of knowledge and understanding of them.

Naturally this neither precludes nor in any way limits the possibility that if any one of these types of claim is valid, the material it furnishes may generate a distinctive and specialised real science, just as our perceptual data give rise to all the various branches of our perceptual-objective science. And the cultivation and development of such a scientific domain within its own frontiers will be as independent of psychology as are physics or geology. But as cognitive or would-be cognitive states or activities any such special types of truth-claim not only belong to psychology also, but they do so first of all because it is the business of the latter to inquire into their precise psychological scope and status, i.e. the experienced characters or marks or relationships or connections which are held to distinguish them and on which their claims rely.

This falls within the particular field of cognitive psychology. However, in addition, as we have noted, all these states or activities have their inevitable place as psychological phenomena in our total psychic context. In that sense we can say that psychology is the fundamental phenomenological or empirical science : everything we can conceive or think of enters *eo ipso* into our psychic life, whatever other status it may have as well. A complete description of our psychic history can leave nothing out and can only at its peril (as regards accuracy and adequacy) neglect to study the relations and connections of any element or part with any and all of the others. In effect, to return to our specific issue, if there are sources and forms of valid knowledge other than those of which we have traced the origin and growth, it is obviously vital to any complete account of our history to show where and how they come in (or are first found), what part their validity plays, how they affect such other psychic modes as feeling and desiring, and how they influence the course of our actions. (Clearly similar questions

F

arise if any of these supposed sources of knowledge are in fact sources of chronic error and delusion ; but in that case, curiously enough, their status as psychological phenomena will be much more readily recognised.) All this, however, can only be ascertained by attending to our psychic history and noting, recording, comparing and generally investigating its phenomena, exactly like any others in their appropriate field. The sole alternative would be to philosophise about them in the traditional way : to start from such ideas as we find circulating in philosophic debate, to take sides about them according to received theories, to argue out their implications, or alleged implications, etc. We know what the results of these processes are, and we have seen how little we can expect any others. If on the other hand we break out of this endless circle of abstract ratiocination and dialectical argument and turn instead to the field of actual occurrence of any recognisable psychological phenomena involved, we shall find ourselves drawn deeper and deeper into the network of the concrete facts, and the result of following their lead and steadfastly learning from them will automatically constitute further empirical—and cumulative—science.

Of course if we do, in the course of building up a complete psychology of knowledge as part of a comprehensive total psychology, identify ways of evolving authentic bodies of knowledge other than our empirical sciences, or for that matter of achieving authentic but isolated pieces of non-perceptual cognition, these will have the double status, both of being psychological and of standing for some independent reality, very much like our empirical sciences themselves. But that follows later ; the first task is to find and describe and circumscribe the various ways, or supposed ways, of " knowing," in their actual place and mode of occurrence in the psychological context. That is an undertaking which can only fall to our comprehensive psychological science.

(5) Without any least pretence to proper appraisal and merely for the sake of illustrating our argument, we may now proceed to glance very summarily over some of the main sources of knowledge or of alleged knowledge, other than empirical learning and its direct derivatives, which have at various times been put forward. We have already enumerated most of them in Chapter V and may repeat the catalogue here, premising only that (*a*) many of them have ill-defined overlaps with one or more of the others, and (*b*) whilst we can broadly distinguish between Groups I and II, the boundary between them is far from clear.

GROUP I : (CLAIMING TRUTH WHOLLY OR CHIEFLY IN THE PERCEPTUAL-PHYSICAL OR PSYCHOLOGICAL WORLD).

(i) Innate or inherited knowledge.
(ii) Instinctive knowledge.
(iii) Intuition.
(iv) Logical inference.
(v) Logical construction.
(vi) Prophecy.
(vii) Veridical or prophetic dreaming.
(viii) Clairvoyance.
(ix) Communication from disembodied spirits, direct or through mediums.
(x) Telepathy.
(xi) Magical or occult knowledge.

GROUP II : (CLAIMING TRUTH WHICH TRANSCENDS BOTH THE ABOVE WORLDS).

(xii) Revelation.
(xiii) Mystical vision.
(xiv) Religious experience.
(xv) Ethical experience.
(xvi) Aesthetic experience.

With regard to Group I it is in most cases obvious that the information claimed as derived from these sources is information which refers either to the psychological world (telepathy, but also, at least in part, instinct and intuition) or to the perceptual-physical one. In some instances the knowledge gained is thought to go partly beyond either of these worlds ; and in at least one, its relation to the perceptual-physical world is equivocal and controversial. But in the main it is plain from the nature of all these cases that the truth-claim is subject to the tests—voluntarily sought or involuntarily suffered—of the actual future course of our objective or perceptual experience ; and we are dealing with the straightforward empirical questions (*a*) whether we can identify information, or apparent information, which has definitely been obtained from one of these non-perceptual sources ; (*b*) how reliable, in the light of actual experiential tests, such information has proved to be.

It is then a matter for detailed inquiry what the answers to these questions are in each type of case. The following comments are only by way of the broadest preliminary sorting out.

(6), Group I : (i) and (ii) " Innate ideas " in the old-fashioned sense in which Locke discussed and rejected them are hardly serious candidates for acceptance today, but in the form of inherited or instinctive information of some kind (implicit or functional or even structural) which does not have to be learnt but under appropriate conditions becomes available to us, it has obvious and reasonable claims to consideration. Something extraordinarily like inherited, unlearnt knowledge (in structural and functional form) is in evidence in many sections of the animal world (specially familiar to most of us in birds, mammals, and insects). It would be surprising rather than otherwise if we had nothing of the kind. But on the other hand such knowledge is certainly not on view with us in manifest and unmistakable guises, like the highly elaborate pre-adapted behaviour patterns of so many other species of animal. If it exists, it is heavily overlaid with learnt information (and modes of action), and extremely difficult to identify, whilst in any case its scope would seem to be very limited. However, there is probably room, in various possible directions, for much more searching experimental investigation than has been given to the subject yet ; what is patent is that it is one for ordinary scientific inquiry. And even if in the end we did solidly establish the existence of significant bodies of inherited or instinctive human knowledge, few people in our day would wish to claim infallible reliability for it ; no doubt many remarkably accurate and successful types of instinctive performance on the part of animals are on record, but there is also ample evidence how readily, if there is any unusual variation in the conditions, such performances can be led astray.

(iii) The claims of a special faculty or power of direct intuition as a source of immediate (unlearnt) knowledge and insight are far more dubious in their nature, and can be regarded as largely discredited. Philosophic discussions of such claims are apt to get caught in the usual inextricable tangling up of questions about word-meanings, questions about the nature and implications of ideas, and questions about facts, so that there rarely emerges a case clear enough for specific examination. And if there does, or if a definite claim is put forward in a non-philosophic context, it is very often possible to show without difficulty that the particular piece of supposed immediate intuitive insight is in fact only a swift implicit inference which can readily be traced back to its learnt elements. Actually most highly trained people proceed habitually in this way in their own field, reading a whole situation by signs which they interpret automatically and without specific consciousness in the light of their accumulated familiarity with and knowledge of the given field (e.g., the " clinical sense " of first-class physicians). And most of us possess a fund of such familiarity and knowledge within the domain of our ordinary experience, in such matters, for instance, as human nature and motives. (But how often such " intuitions " go astray !)

All the foregoing does not prove that there may not after all be left a residuum of genuine knowledge of the type of immediate unlearnt intuition—even though still further scrutiny *might* reduce this to our Groups (i) and (ii). But again there is no way of surely establishing the facts except by close empirical inquiry into actual alleged cases and their different categories, circumstances and conditions, if only in order to eliminate the possibility of immediate implicit inferences, such as we can so often demonstrate. Whilst as far as reliability is concerned, the record of many claimed applications of intuition could hardly be worse, and sheer fairness to this potential source of unlearnt insight demands that judgment about it should be suspended until the existence of genuinely intuitive information has incontestably been shown.

(7), (iv) The case of logical inference is obviously totally different. Here there is no doubt about the facts. They are not indeed—as modern logicians have brought out—anywhere near as simple as the Aristotelian type of logic assumed. If all inference were syllogistic, on the Aristotelian pattern, we should not need to postulate more than the primitive expectation-situation discussed in Chapter III, and could evolve all later forms of articulated inference from this. Much can in fact be done on these lines and certainly all the main classes of Aristotelian syllogistic inference can be thus derived (including its various auxiliary forms). Moreover, with an effort most if not all of the more modern types of relational inference could be forced into the same pattern and equally developed from one sort of expectation-situation or another.

But the true interest of knowledge demands sharp emphasis on distinctions, at least as much as the uncovery of common features. It seems important therefore to acknowledge, at any rate as a provisionally autonomous fact, that we possess extensive powers of obtaining new information by inferences of markedly different orders from that of the applicative or subsumptive syllogism inherent in our typical expectation-situations. Modern logic has brought to light the many diverse ways in which we can combine two suitably related pieces of information to yield a third, which is not merely a case, or class of cases, under one of the first two, but an authentic new addition to our knowledge, of the same order of value. (Anything that has property A, has property B. Anything with property B, has property C. Therefore anything with property A, has property C. Or : event A is always followed by event B ; event B is always followed by event C ; therefore event A is always followed by event C. Or : event A is always followed within five minutes by event B ; event B is always followed within five minutes by event C. Therefore event A is always followed within ten minutes by event C, etc., etc.)

These powers of combining suitable pieces of existing knowledge to generate new information offer an extremely interesting field for further *empirical psychological* inquiry. They have so far been mostly left to logicians, whose concern with them has naturally been circumscribed by their strictly formal approach.[1]

We cannot do much more here than to note the possibilities of the theme. The sole directly relevant points from our angle are, first : that there are plenty of pit-falls in the inferential use of many if not all of these relations—pitfalls which are demonstrated in the accustomed way by our actually finding ourselves misled, i.e. confronted with a concrete (perceived) situation which is different from what we had inferred (and so expected). And secondly that in any case, quite apart from the pitfalls attaching to the relations themselves, none of our inferred new information can claim a greater reliability than that of both or all of the beliefs related. In so far as any or all of these are themselves empirically learnt pieces of information, they are liable, like any others, to be wrong, or to have latent elements of error in them. And indeed the new combination of two or more previously separate beliefs may well *bring out* any latent defects or limitations in one or another of them, so that the new piece of inferred information is often in peculiar need of empirical test and confirmation. But it does very commonly receive this, and relational inference is thus without a doubt a potent and invaluable source of information, even of a general kind, which is new and yet has not had to be learnt from experience (or socially communicated). However, it is no more than an auxiliary instrument, even if a very powerful one, and it

---

[1] A more apparent than real exception is provided by the work of Professor Spearman, who saw the importance, for a proper *psychology* of cognition, of the general theme of the eduction of relations and correlates. Unfortunately, however, his approach is completely non-genetic, and his treatment of relations particularly scholastic and unilluminating.

remains mainly if not wholly subject to the test or the challenge of further primary (chiefly perceptual) experience. The possible exception is of course that of new information inferred from prior knowledge (if there is any) which (*a*) has not itself been learnt from experience, but (*b*) is of a kind, or comes from a source, already established as completely reliable or infallible. Even that would still leave the question whether the inferential process might not introduce some fallibility of its own, and this raises the issue how we can distinguish inferential relations which can lead us astray from such as cannot. However, by and large the problem comes back at this point to that of the true sources, if any, of unlearnt and completely assured primary or factual knowledge capable, *inter alia*, of providing the premises for logical inference. The contribution which the latter as such can make to this is limited, at the best, to those auxiliaries of knowledge, the relations of overlap, etc., by which different pieces of information can be linked together.

(v) The foregoing comes close to, and perhaps encroaches upon, our next category, logically constructed knowledge. The latter description is itself controversial and possibly question-begging for the topic I have chiefly in mind here, viz., mathematics. And this, in whatever way it should be classified, is so important and difficult a theme that it seems best to postpone it till we have completed our general survey, and to give it somewhat closer consideration at that stage.

(8), (vi) to (xi) For our restricted purpose here, we can collect together all these suggested sources of knowledge not learnt either directly or indirectly by the ordinary processes of experience. They mostly belong, or at least have belonged in the past, in greater or less degree, to the obscure and uncertain world which we vaguely call that of the supernatural. They have considerable overlaps with one another, and also some overlap with our Group II. But on the other hand many people would make a sharp distinction between several of them and the rest, and also between the status of some of them today and that of all of them prior to say the second half of the nineteenth century. As a result of the work done by the Society for Psychical Research, it would be contended that some of these sources of knowledge were now scientifically established. In the case of telepathy the claim would be endorsed by a number of general psychologists ; some who would indeed maintain that it was the one element of fact underlying, and in the main accounting for, the other merely fanciful beliefs. On the other hand most of them would also insist that it was a very limited element of fact solely showing that we could get *psychological* information (information about elements of other people's states of mind) without needing to pass through the usual perceptual media of communication.—In the case of prophetic dreaming it has likewise been claimed that the facts have been established by ordinary scientific methods and their accepted canons, and can be so tested and confirmed.

We are not seeking here to examine or evaluate these claims. We acknowledge that some of them are today on a different footing from others, and our sole reasons for bringing them together are their historical association with one another and their various overlaps. In fact these claims only concern us for the moment from one angle. Their very history of the last decades brings out that what they seek to make good is their validity in our established objective world. They fully accept the evidence and tests of this, and have particularly sought to secure the status and credit of regular empirical scientific knowledge.

It is obvious that if that goal had been completely attained, these now accredited modes of cognition would at once become an integral and most important part of empirical psychology. (That is, in one aspect ; prophetic dreams, for example, might also have their contributions to make to all sorts of other bodies of knowledge : perhaps even to a new and odd science of their own—the science of futurity as such !)

Nothing could be more vital for any true scientific picture of the scope and significance of our psychic life, and of its structure and laws. We need not, however, elaborate the theme, because so far this fundamental accession to scientific psychology can hardly be said to have taken place yet. Scientific psychologists still fight shy of most so-called " psychic " phenomena ; by a curious twist even the scientific, or would-be scientific investigation of their reality and import has been largely taken up by amateurs from other fields. And the apparently positive results have been less convincing than they might have been just because these clearly psychological investigations have been carried out for the most part by persons who both lacked proper psychological training and background, *and* were unaware of the need for these. (One would like to hear some of the physicists who have constituted themselves psychic researchers comment on psychologists without any training or background in physics who constituted themselves researchers in advanced physical phenomena.)

There are indeed many grounds for psychological criticism of the supposedly scientific " psychic " research carried out by non-psychologists, and thus for reserve about the apparent results claimed by them. The latter have moreover remained curiously isolated and merely repetitive, instead of cumulative in the way so characteristic of all other empirical scientific inquiry. It is therefore still reasonable to view most of these " paranormal " modes of cognition as at the best not finally established yet ; and even about telepathy the last critical word may not as yet have been said. In truth, some of the cognitive claims which occupy psychical researchers can scarcely be regarded so far as more than marginal question-marks. The whole range of so-called " psychic phenomena " should probably receive more thorough attention than it has done hitherto from fully trained psychologists with the right background. Meanwhile, all these alleged special sources of knowledge are at any rate recognised here as possibilities. They cannot indeed alter the broad picture of our main learning processes and their results as set out earlier, though they may mean that it is incomplete. And this may have a bearing on its ultimate or philosophic interpretation. The one thing which is clear, however, is that the specific consideration of the reality, and if this can be established, of the various relationships and con-sequences of any or all of the above phenomena is not a matter for philosophy ; it is one for " psychic research " in what should be the correct sense of the phrase, i.e., for empirical psychological investigation.

(9) If we turn now to Group II we come to believed sources of knowledge which mainly, if not wholly, claim reference to an order of reality transcending not only our subjective-psychological but also our perceptual-objective world. These sources are therefore regarded as, at least in principle, not subject to any perceptual tests. Perceptual evidence held to testify to their validity is not indeed disclaimed (in fact as regards " revelation " in all its earlier forms, such evidence is largely relied upon), but any perceptual factors pointing in the opposite direction are either interpreted away, or lead to a rebuttal in principle of the relevance of per-ceptual data as such.

We have already made our appropriate general comments on this group, and can add little by way of specific annotation with-out going too far out of our course. We can distinguish between revelation and mystical vision (xii and xiii) on the one hand, and religious, ethical and aesthetic experience (xiv—xvi) on the

F*

other, in so far as the former claim their own overriding sphere, transcending even philosophy. The latter sub-group, by way of contrast, tends to be a typical philosophic preoccupation—but one which, very curiously, emphasises its psychological basis in "experience" whilst nevertheless it sharply repudiates any dependence on mere empirical psychology.

However, even (xii) and (xiii) raise, as we have seen, inescapable psychological questions. If there can be such a thing as false soi-disant "revelation" and false soi-disant "mystical vision," i.e., fantasies or delusions or errors wrongly thought to be what they are not, what is the way in which we can distinguish between the real thing and such mirages or false images of it? (*A*) What *constitutes* "truth" as against "falsity" in revelations and visions (of which the content expressly claims to transcend our ordinary visible world)? What do we mean here by these contrasted characters or descriptions? (*B*) By what specific criteria can we decide in a particular case which kind, the genuine or the spurious, we are dealing with? ((*A*) Should of course lead straight on to (*B*). What we are seeking is any set of marks, relationships or experiential connections which will enable us to distinguish between truth and error, as we have seen we can do in the case of beliefs referring to our perceptual-objective world.

These are once more partly psycho-linguistic questions, partly substantive psychological ones, before they are anything else. When they have been successfully answered on that level, the way should be open to a greater, trans-psychological world, very much as the same treatment of perception leads out into the physical world.

But first there is the psychological issue, the question of the manner in which we can discriminate between what is " merely " my state, and what indeed begins for me as such but then goes beyond this. We have already noted that the answer, if it is *not* to be in terms of our perceptual-objective world, has always hither-to proved extraordinarily difficult and elusive. Any discussions on the subject have in fact only led into the familiar philosophic circle of verbal, conceptual and factual issues endlessly sliding into one another and leading nowhere but into endlessly self-repeating controversy. Nevertheless, it behoves us here to leave fully open the possibility that the human experiences or reported experiences we call revelation and mystic vision may, at least in some cases, have a veridical significance of their own which it may be most important to appreciate ; and what we are suggesting is precisely that, if this is so, the one way of establishing it is not to regard the problem as one for philosophy, but to treat it seriously and soberly and specifically as first of all a psychological question, or rather a set of such questions, as above set out. That the status and bearings of these experiences are in turn not irrelevant to our endeavours to build up an adequate empirical psychology has, since William James, been plain to at least the more catholic among psychologists.

(10) With regard to (xiv–xvi), the usual background of assumption is of course that empirical psychology is or may be interested in what are held to be certain specific modes or orders of experience as *psychic occurrences*, but philosophy alone is concerned with the question of anything they may involve beyond themselves, any distinctive order of *reality* or *actuality* which they may disclose or point to. And many philosophers have in fact held that it can be shown that one or another of these types of experience, or even all three of them, do point to their distinctive orders of reality, either analogously to the way in which our perceptual-cognitive experience does—or far more truly and dependably so. There has indeed even been the view that ethical experience discloses real ethical properties or characters or qualities of either persons or actions or states in precisely the same (strictly perceptual) way as vision discloses qualities of colour, shape, etc., and as our other perceptual modes yield their characteristic objective correlates.

But unfortunately actual philosophic discussion, even though this unwonted stress on the concrete contents of experience as experience provides it with a far more solid foundation than it usually commands, soon loses itself again in its accustomed dialectical difficulties. And the only way out is once more to reverse the initial false and arbitrary assumption about the limits of empirical psychology and to start with the right psycho-linguistic and substantively psychological questions. What is the sense of " reality " or " actuality " in which we believe—if we believe—that either religious or ethical or aesthetic experience discloses a reality beyond its own (subjective) occurrence ? And one as real as, or more real than, but certainly different from that opened up by perceptual experience ? What is the experiential content, or what are the experiential distinguishing marks, of this special and distinctive reality ? And what, therefore, are the criteria by which we can (or could) decide whether any particular soi-disant religious or ethical or aesthetic experience is authentic and veridical—

since patently there are many so-styled which we all claim the right to reject ?

The difficulties of finding satisfactory answers to these questions are at best very great. Yet in this field where we are dealing with vast complexes of psychological facts, " mere " psychology may have much more to contribute than we allow for if we too rashly take adult religious or ethical or aesthetic experience at its face-value and address our questions to it as it stands. Each of these modes of experience has a long history in us, partly individual, partly superimposed social. It can safely be said that the full psychological story as we are now able to trace it, especially in the case of our religious and moral experience, has never yet been taken into account. It represents at least as intricate a pattern of multiple and cumulative trains of psychic happenings as, say, the development of our notion of and belief in causality ; indeed this and the course of our cognitive experiences generally have had a large part to play in the growth of our moral ideas. If these factors and the full light shed on our affective-conative history by psycho-analysis are properly considered, it may turn out that there is little room left for any further question. The very notion of some objective reality which is specifically apprehended by or in our ethical or religious experience may owe most of its appearance of reasonableness to the obvious inability of past *single* psychological explanations of that experience to account adequately for it. And if in fact it proves impossible to formulate either any distinctive definition of or any criteria for " reality " or " objectivity " to provide a separate realm of reference and control for our supposed ethical or religious apprehension, our picture would be consistent and complete.

But all this must here be left hypothetical.[1] We need not, from our angle of approach, reject the theoretical possibility that this or that more or less distinct mode of experience may have its own special contribution of knowledge to make to the sum-total of our information about a real world (or worlds) independent of our " knowing " states. All we can say is that first of all we must make sure that we have the full psychological story of that mode of experience as it has come to be what it is. And that is a matter for empirical psychology, not for philosophy. It is no better than an empirical psychological blunder (completely disregarding the nature of our psychological material) to treat the current form of

---

[1] I hope to deal with the genetic psychology of our ethical beliefs (with its interesting parallels to and divergences from our physical beliefs) in a subsequent volume.

a particular mode of experience, which is in fact a complex historical product, as a simple *given* reality in its own right, from which we can draw conclusions to some *corresponding* simple reality outside it.

(11) Finally, we may now turn again to the difficult and complex theme of our sub-group (v)—or our system of mathematical constructions, inferences and theorems. This, as we are all aware, has long been regarded as the ideal and perfect exemplar of what all science should be, and has led to the fond assumption that philosophic insight should, and could, be secured by similar methods setting out from similar starting-points. Here there has in fact appeared to be a process by which a great body of authentic knowledge (dependably true beliefs) has been built up by the mind's own resources from principles and data which themselves seemed to owe little if anything to the world of perceptual experience, by procedures which owed even less, with results which were so intrinsically assured that testing or verification in the perceptual world appeared to be not only unnecessary but irrelevant. In so far, however, as situations arose—as they constantly did—in which mathematical knowledge could be applied to that world, one could take it completely for granted that it would be verified, and in fact it always was.[1]

Hence all that was believed to be necessary in *any* field of thought was to start from equally clear principles and properly defined ideas, and to use the same rigorous method of reasoning, whereupon one could, as a matter of course, expect to construct similar bodies of true conclusions, or assured knowledge.

It has not in fact worked out that way ; on the evidence of results alone, the case, as we have already observed, is clearly one of a false transfer of beliefs by analogy. The actual history of all the *philosophic* attempts to build up knowledge on this assumption shows that the supposed analogy must be invalid, and that this is an instance where, in the light of their breakdown, we must reconsider our previous beliefs and, as far as may be necessary, revise and correct them.

---

[1] It might be said—and has been—that we should never *allow* a mathematical proposition to be falsified, because if it appeared to be, we should regard it as inapplicable. If one drop of water added to another drop made not two but a single (bigger) drop, this would not signify that one plus one were ever other than two, but only that we were talking of the idea of one and the idea of one, and the idea of addition, not of what would happen if two physical entities were brought into contact (or even proximity !). But this merely means that mathematical propositions are only held to be true in any given context if certain specified conditions are fulfilled. The same applies to all other propositions, and it remains a fact that *within* the specified conditions, mathematical propositions are never falsified.

Yet that leaves us, as always, with the question on our hands how it is that our generalisation holds good in its original field : mathematics remains with us, with all the apparent characteristics described above, and we have more than ever to seek to understand what its own (so far unique) success depends upon.

We are here only concerned again with acknowledging the problem, rather than with trying to establish any particular solution, and we must once more conclude that it is one for the appropriate empirical science, in this case the empirical psychology of knowledge ; like any other anomaly, or seeming anomaly, within the latter's field, and like any problem of a seeming anomaly in any other empirical-scientific field.

That of course is a view which will be regarded as nonsensical, not merely by traditional philosophers but still more by present-day philosophic mathematicians or mathematical philosophers. These latter indeed, in the name of their more rigorous logic, reject without ceremony the ordinary philosophic fumblings and gropings about the nature and place of mathematical truths, but they would rebut even more forcibly the preposterous idea that empirical psychologists could have any business in this field. The fundamental reasons why so unacceptable a view must nevertheless be maintained have already been supplied by the whole tenor of the present essay ; but on the other hand it must at once be conceded that in a highly specialised domain such as that of mathematics, the empirical psychologist who is to do justice to it must also command a high degree of mathematical competence. Since I have no pretensions to this, I must in the main be content with the merely negative and extraneous evidence already adduced that mathematics is a special case. But it remains a case—and that is the important point—of a specific human activity in the cognitive field, which must be investigated against the total background of that field and of our other activities in it ; in effect, as a problem of the determining conditions which allow local success where apparently similar activities applied elsewhere produce failure.

(12) There are, however, some supplementary points which seem worth making. Curiously enough, although for modern mathematician-philosophers the present approach is anathema, their own most current view of the nature of mathematics is one which, if it is correct, fits in very well with the picture of the main movement of scientific learning and knowledge offered here. I refer to the familiar contemporary thesis that mathematical

" knowledge " is essentially tautological. In that case our problem disappears ; there is no longer any anomaly, for mathematics is not strictly speaking knowledge at all, but a mere auxiliary technique, a means of ordering, marshalling and manipulating knowledge. It is based on conventional rules which obviously have to be mastered and properly carried out if the technique is to work, but it is nothing that can in any way claim to rival the authentic body of objective truth which we can only gather by continuous and cumulative apprenticeship to the external world.

Even a tyro in mathematics can broadly appreciate the way in which this result is reached from a consideration of the meaning of algebra, which so plainly appears as the fundamental form of mathematical procedure. Nevertheless there are points at which a student of the psychological data and settings of knowledge may legitimately feel the lack of any psychological grasp or background on the part of most of the mathematician-philosophers advocating the above view, and the effects of their assumption that these things cannot possibly be relevant. For better or worse, they are dealing throughout with psychological phenomena with a psychological history ; phenomena, moreover, which form part of a single larger psychic context and of a single comprehensive psychic history. For the development of mathematical ideas along their own lines in their own field, these facts can no doubt be disregarded, but not for the understanding of their place in the wider cognitive context, and of their relation to the rest.

Thus we might ask for a start, from a psycho-linguistic angle, whether the notion of tautology can really bear the weight which the above theory places on it—and how far it remains the same notion if that weight is put on it ? If we take other tautologies, of all the kinds that have given the term its original meaning, where shall we find any that have undergone developments or had consequences comparable with those of mathematics—where shall we find any, indeed, that have any sort of major function or value at all ? Mathematics seems even more of an anomaly as a system of tautologies than as a body of objective knowledge ! Taken in their ordinary sense tautologies are the barrenest and emptiest plays with words, from which one cannot imagine anything useful emerging. We should not even use the term normally for the contents of foreign language dictionaries or specialised glossaries, which do have a genuine though extremely limited function, but in very virtue of that fact are regarded as something different from " mere " tautologies. It is plain, therefore, that something very odd must have happened to the normal meaning of the term when it is applied to what is so obviously—at the least—the most powerful and fruitful of all the *instruments* at the service of cumulative knowledge. Is the word " tautology " when so employed as revealing as it purports to be, or is it now merely misleading? Has the question of the nature of mathematics thus been really answered—or only begged?

At any rate the psychological student contemplating the historical and current functioning of mathematical knowledge can hardly feel very happy or illuminated over the choice of this particular term, and the analogy it implies, as the sole and sufficient key to its significance. It certainly achieves the object of separating mathematics radically from all genuine knowledge, but *if* it retains any considerable part of its original sense, it does seem to overshoot its mark. (If it does not, why use it? And *what is really being said?*) Thus the psychologist who wants to understand what mathematics is and what has made it so immensely important and fruitful in the history of all scientific knowledge, as well as of most successful human action, can hardly resist the fear that the " tautological " theory is not very searching or very profound psychology, or very adequate to or commensurate with the phenomenon for which it seeks to account. He can see that there is something significant in it, but he cannot help being afraid that it may be rather too simple and easy, and may go much too far. It seems desirable, therefore, from his point of view, to recognise at least the possibility that there may be a genuine and unsolved problem left on our hands after all. And indeed he can find something very like authentic empirical support for this. Geometrical propositions, for instance, can be verified in specific instances in the perceptual world in precisely the same way as any other ordinary expectations, or applications of an empirical general proposition to a new case. And it seems even that the verification can break down in a similar fashion under conditions different enough from our normal ones, though in the latter such propositions have a far higher degree of dependability than most of our ordinary beliefs.—The same applies, though perhaps with rather more room for theoretical argument, in the case of arithmetical propositions, and even (at a further remove) of algebraical ones. The appearance, at this last stage, of mere tautology is very strong, but if these tautologies, unlike any others, can be translated into specific perceptual predictions or anticipations, and duly verified . . . . .?

Furthermore there are properties of perceptual objects and objective entities which we actually find, and which might not have been there, but which seem to correspond in a special way to the bodies of knowledge, or soi-disant knowledge, we call mathematics. These properties are of a distinctive and peculiar type ; not positive characteristics which we discover in things, so much as susceptibilities to actions which can be *performed* on or with them ; actions which *we* can usually perform and which mostly have the further distinctive characteristic of not materially changing them. Objects can be aggregated and separated, individually and in groups ; they can be superimposed on one another and compared in this respect, or contained in one another and compared that way. These are passive properties which, on the one hand, usually affect the objects in no other way, but on the other lend themselves peculiarly to operation by us, both in the actual perceptual world and in thought. When we work with objects in this way in our thought, we can simplify them down to the completest constancy and uniformity and bare " thereness," as carriers of those properties ; and that in turn makes the possibilities for such mental manipulation all the wider, easier, and more varied.—Furthermore, there is an empirical history of gradual development of our recognition of these properties, of our progressive use of them, and of our increasing exploitation of just the above wider scope which we find offered by them ; all remarkably similar to the history of all our other advances in discovery and knowledge, skills and powers.

The foregoing suggests, as at least a conceivable alternative to the tautological view (an alternative which has indeed had its advocates before), that mathematics may be a genuine but singular and circumscribed type of knowledge, based on such properties as the above, plus our discovery of all the patterns they give rise to in the empirical world and all the further ones which we can endlessly build up from them in our own thought. It is not difficult to show, on that basis, how mathematical knowledge comes to possess the extraordinary instrumental fruitfulness and power which we actually find. This approach cannot be further pursued here, and is indeed not of great value without the backing of a degree of proficiency in the whole field of mathematics which I cannot claim. The important points, which clearly stand out even without specialised proficiency, are these : (i) mathematics appears to represent the one unquestionable case of (non-psychological) knowledge not built up from perception nor in need of perceptual tests—in fact a vast and immensely solid structure of authentic non-empirical science ; but it is in truth either not knowledge at all or else a peculiar limited form of this, easily segregated from the rest and dependent on very special conditions. (ii) Either way, its great role in our cognitive history has been that of an auxiliary instrument (however indispensable and fruitful and powerful) in the growth of our empirical knowledge or science. (iii) In that role it has been fully subject to the demands and vicissitudes of empirical inquiry and empirical (perceptual) tests : the matter to which mathematical methods or mathematical results have been applied has always superimposed on these its own empirical conditions and limitations. What we have already noted in connection with our sub-group (iv) (logically inferred information), holds equally as regards every kind of mathematical construction, the moment this is given any concrete empirical or perceptual content. This manifest parallel is indeed only to be expected if, as has been insisted by the most eminent modern logicians and mathematical philosophers, logic and mathematics are at bottom one. But whether or not that proposition is both fully clear and fully established, there can be no doubt about their comparable instrumental functions in the growth of our empirical knowledge of our world, and their common subordination throughout the field of the latter to the primacy of factual investigation and factual tests. The latter thus once more retain the last word. And we may insist again that for all the reasons we have shown, they do so also as regards the very problem of the ultimate sources, roots and scope of those specific psychological activities, our logical and mathematical operations themselves.

(13) What we have done so far in this section has been to try to complete the picture of what, on our approach, the philosophic theory of knowledge is *not* concerned with. Any and every specific problem about the scope and conditions of our learning and knowing states and activities is first of all a matter of specific factual inquiry in the right context and against the right background of our cognitive psychology as a whole, set in turn within the scheme of the widest general psychology we know—a psychology that takes into account the full breadth and the full depth of the cumulative experience-histories which make up our psychic lives. This applies to the problem of truth and falsity, that of the external world and of causality, the problem of explanation, and those of all the various special forms and sources of knowledge and truth, or alleged knowledge and truth, from intuition to

revelation, from telepathy to ethical or mystical experience, and from magic to mathematics.

What then, on this view, is left for the philosophic theory of knowledge? It may perhaps appear to have been suggested here at an earlier stage that empirical psychology surveys the facts, and then, but only then, philosophic epistemology considers the problems. Any appearance to this effect has, however, already been corrected : the problems left over by the facts, as we know them so far, are in the first place challenges to continued *factual* investigation, and invitations to try to extend our knowledge further and more deeply by more searching *observations and comparisons*, together with the closer study of relations, connections, conditions and interdependences. It may indeed be that when we have tried everything we can within the factual field, we shall still have on our hands problems with which we can do nothing more along this line of approach and which we can then only recognise as of the special kind we describe as philosophic or ultimate. But there is no reason, except the self-repeating circle of philosophic tradition, why we should behave differently in the particular phenomenal territory we call psychological from the way we do in all the others (actually no less psychological in their primary content for us) which we classify as physical. We realise throughout the latter that problems arising out of the known facts must be pursued by fuller extensions of our knowledge of the facts, and by more penetrating attempts to lay bare their interrelations and structures. And *not* by breaking off physical, or chemical, or astronomic or geological inquiry, and handing over the subject to philosophers, so that they may try to settle our physical or chemical or astronomic or geological mysteries by setting to work, through logical analysis or dialectical debate, on the pure ideas involved.

This does not in truth ever occur to anybody because, once we establish the right orientation to the controlling field of fact, it is so clear that we can and must go on following the lead of the latter as far as ever it will take us. We cannot think profitably without knowing our full facts, and that always means more facts, and not only extensively but also intensively. Only if we remain so effectively caught up in the trammels of philosophic debate as to disregard the appropriate fact-field altogether, can it seem plausible to us to treat specific local problems of our experience as inherently philosophic ones, which can solely be dealt with by philosophic analysis and argument.

What then, once more, *is* left to the philosophic theory of know-ledge ? We have eliminated, as we have seen, specific cognitive problems, at any rate so long as there remains the possibility of further factual inquiry and factual learning. (And for that there is the amplest scope.) But even less can we say that there are any distinctive and superior *methods* by which problems too refractory for an empirical scientific approach can be brought nearer to a solution by means of philosophic attack. Philosophy has indeed its distinctive methods ; its main past difference from empirical science has consisted in this fact, only partly masked by apparent differences of subject-matter. Driven by empirical science out of virtually all the physical world, philosophy has concentrated on those parts of the psychological domain in which its procedures have not, or not yet, been challenged. Yet in fact these are, as we have urged, wholly a muddle and largely a mistake. They are based on the assumption that we can arrive at true knowledge out of our own (existing) notional resources either by abstract thought or by dialectical debate, applied to abstract ideas in a vacuum. Misled, as we have seen, by a quite inappropriate extension of the mathematical analogy to fields in which none of the conditions of success of mathematical operations are fulfilled, philosophic thought has become caught up in a complex, self-renewing vicious system of interlocking circular arguments about implications of ideas, meanings of words, truth of views, criteria of truth, views about criteria of truth, meanings of such views, and so on and on. Philosophic method is what we should expect from its fruits, and its fruits are what we should expect from such a method.

By the same token, scientific procedure is *not* something parallel but different, applicable as it were in its own field but nowhere else. On our view, it is simply a breakaway from the whole cycle of false assumptions and confusions which so effectively sterilises our philosophic thought. It is the discovery of the right kind of control under which we can gain orderly, stable and progressive knowledge, wherever it is applied. Its character, most summarily described as that of fact-control, is actually that of control by the appropriate field of primary experience, secured by submissive attention directed to the appropriate primary-experience-foci. Under the auspices of sustained submission to such fact-control we build up detailed procedures and canons, directions and aims which are everywhere found to yield compre-hensive, coherent and powerful bodies of knowledge. And the " scientific method " thus developed is simply our one *general* method of achieving "science," i.e., tested and cumulative knowledge—the one procedure which has been found applicable and dependable in every field of experience in which it has been tried. We have agreed that there may be other means of securing knowledge ; but if so, they would appear to be at best local and limited, and the claims of most of them have yet to be properly investigated. In any event there is a very strong case for holding that the only way in which we can give distinctive meaning to such claims is by reference to *some appropriate mode* of fact-control (independent of themselves) by which they can be verified—or falsified. From some such criterion as this we do not seem to be able to get away. And quite apart from anything else, the distinctive procedures we adopt in philosophic reflection and argument cannot be regarded as serious claimants ; they obviously do not lead to stable and cumulative knowledge, and they can easily be shown to be riddled with defects and confusions.

(14) We therefore find ourselves more than ever with our question on our hands : what scope does there remain for the philosophic theory of knowledge ? But now it seems as if the issue is really wider than that : what scope does there remain for philosophy as a whole ? We have suggested that our only established, generally valid method of inquiry is that of empirical science, which is typically one of local inquiry under local fact-control and which generates (or expands) specific empirical science wherever it is applied. Does this not come back then to the familiar nineteenth century thesis that philosophy has once and for all been superseded by empirical science ? With the only modification that empirical psychology in general and the empirical psychology of knowledge in particular are left in a master position, because the former is concerned with the whole of experience, and the latter with the investigation of every claimed source of knowledge ? Modern logical positivism would, I believe, differ from such a point of view only in not conceding any special key status to psychology, and in retaining (largely in its stead) a *transitional* cleaning-up role for philosophy in the shape of logical analysis. But this would then be little else than a role of self-dissolution through the clearing up of all the aberrations and muddles of language which have given rise to the pseudo-questions of metaphysics—problems with a misleading appearance of sense, which are really nonsense.

The foregoing is not, however, the view which is suggested here. There is a definite, though a somewhat paradoxical place left for philosophy, which follows directly from the character and the limitations of empirical science. The latter is essentially *local* and progressive, turning one after another tract of our primary experience into a specific but unfinished body of knowledge. And that then leaves us with a vast deal which goes beyond the scope of any individual empirical science, and by the same token beyond that of the mere sum of such sciences. There is, for a start, our experience as a whole, as a single history, but a history still in process. There is also the current synthesis of the separate pictures of all our different empirical sciences—but again as a synthesis of pictures all still in the making and each at a different level of incompleteness and in a different stage of growth. And there is furthermore the unquestionable fact that our empirical sciences do not by any means cover the whole ground of our experience, firstly because portions of it have barely begun to be explored scientifically, and secondly because much of it (e.g., of our feeling-life) is so inherently fluid and elusive and individual that scientific method, which depends on a clearly shaped repeatableness, or at the least repetition, of experiences, has little chance of securing any purchase on it.

Obviously none of these factors, taken on its merits, affords any particular prospect or hope of super-empirical *knowledge* ; on the contrary, as far as they go, they point away from this. They do nothing to invalidate the conclusion that the only method on which we can in general rely for the acquisition of any desired information or insight is that of empirical-scientific investigation : the above facts simply represent the limits of what this has so far been able to reach. Nevertheless it also remains true that we cannot be content with this. We cannot help straining at the leash and wanting something more, something different, something more satisfying and more final—more satisfying, in effect, because more final. Whether it is answerable or not, we cannot help *experiencing the question* whether we can say anything about our experience as a whole ; whether we can conclude anything from it, or interpret it, or make sense of it. Alternatively we may raise the same issue about the present sum of our empirical scientific knowledge, plus the further question whether any such total interpretation is at least *compatible* with all those elements or aspects of our experience (including any forms of unlearnt knowledge which we believe to be established) which do not form part of any organised empirical science, or anyhow do not do so yet.

(15) It is far from clear that such questions are capable of any

answer, and it seems inevitable that they cannot be answered with any certainty or finality, given our still growing knowledge within a wider history which is itself still in progress. Yet the issues arise and we cannot avoid, nor is there any reason why we should avoid, considering them. They are the proper theme of philosophy, and if we did not already have this recognised name for our widest strivings for the integration and interpretation of all our experience-world, we should sooner or later need to invent one with just that scope. We have in fact to acknowledge the time-honoured meaning and task of philosophy. We eliminate only the false assumption that it has some method of its own, more searching and more efficacious than that by which we discover and test and build up our local truths. It must be content with the self-same procedure and canons, and it has everything to gain by discarding its merely pre-scientific bad habits. And besides getting rid of our traditional philosophic circle of defective data and inadequate logic, we must add, as we have seen, the inescapable limitation which the flaws of philosophic method have so readily allowed it to ignore but which is the one pervasive refrain of our whole knowledge and our whole experience : the fact that any total reading we may essay must jump the unknown degree of incompleteness of our evidence ; the fact that the growth of our knowledge and the process of our history are still going on.

What all this points to as regards both the aims and the status of philosophy is that, except for its far vaster scale, it is essentially comparable to the pursuit of comprehensive explanatory hypotheses—the survey and appraisal of any already in the field, and the endeavour, if none seems to fit all the facts, to think either of some variation that might do so or of some quite different and better solution—within the domain of any of the separate empirical sciences. There are of course new problems and special pitfalls when this approach is applied to the whole of our experience ; doubts whether we are not pressing the very notion of explanation beyond what it will bear, and the certainty that, for the reasons we have already emphasised, our conclusions can at the best only be *speculative*. We cannot develop this theme fully here, but at any rate our approach is here again in harmony with what has been widely recognised throughout the centuries as the distinctive character and limitation of philosophy.

The particular feature of our view is merely its demand that the notions both of explanation and of speculation shall be taken more seriously, examined more carefully, and developed more

fully than has usually been done in the past. " Explanatory "
theories or hypotheses can only be drawn from the material of our
experience ; they consist essentially of taking some known and
familiar process or relation or characteristic or property, imaginatively extending this or transferring it to a new field, and showing
how it could lead to ranges of facts which have not previously been
brought into relation with it. The hypothesis becomes probable in
the measure in which it proves capable of (*a*) thus *illuminating* wide
ranges of known facts (on the assumption that it is true) (*b*) pointing to previously unknown ones which are then actually found
(*c*) being directly verified as a " true cause " (or real state of
affairs), once it is suitably looked for, in a representative range of
those cases which, in so far as correct, it is able to illuminate. But
all these tests depend on the hypothesis having a definite shape
and content, from which determinate consequences follow ; and
if there are several alternatives in the field, they must each have
its own *different* shape and content, from which—at least at some
point—*different* determinate consequences follow.   That these
shapes and contents are always in fact drawn from our previous
experience and knowledge can be shown without difficulty in
the case of all our empirical scientific explanatory theories or
hypotheses.

When now we try to form such hypotheses for the whole
breadth and diversity of our experience, and at the same time have
to allow for its inevitable gaps and unevennesses of development,
as well as its inherently unfinished character, it seems clear that
we cannot hope to establish a higher status for our ventures than
that of speculations.   And in these circumstances we can only
extract the maximum of virtue out of our necessity if we
leave every door wide open for the utmost possible variety and
imaginativeness and boldness in our speculations.   The need for
this is indeed impressed on us, if we start with an open mind at all,
by the manifest breakdowns and failures of all the easy and
natural philosophic interpretative hypotheses we find in the field.
Our early experience suggests naïve anthropomorphic world-
views that soon come into conflict with all the main tenor of the
world which our advancing further knowledge encounters. But
some of this very knowledge may presently seem to suggest even
more strongly than before, though on a higher level, a great
designing and planning and ordering intelligence behind our
given scheme of things ; only to run into further difficulties which
take much or most of the bloom off that promising hypothesis.

Moreover it turns out that various totally different suppositions can also account for many and perhaps all the facts that appeared to call for the first one. Metaphysical philosophers have therefore tried diverse bolder appeals to analogies from other parts of our experience to provide a suggested underlying pattern for all the rest : pantheistic, monadological, absolute idealistic, materialistic, etc. But the propounders of each such view have in turn suffered, as well as inflicted, damaging criticism, usually on grounds of vagueness, shiftingness and self-contradiction in addition to palpable failure to cope with various obstinate sets of factors or aspects of our experience.

This long history of mainly unprogressive strife may provide good reasons for giving up a hopeless enterprise ; and a strong case may be built up for the view that—quite apart from avoidable shortcomings and aberrations of method—the hopelessness of the enterprise is inherent in what it tries to do. Yet that is itself an outcome of philosophic consideration of the problem and no ground whatever for laying down dogmatically in advance that there is no problem to be considered. In fact such a conclusion should in its turn, on our premises, be held only as a working hypothesis, perfectly compatible with the utmost interest in and encouragement of every imaginable further endeavour to suggest new possibilities for speculative exploration. For the question still and always remains on our hands : we find ourselves involved in this history of our own experience, of human experience, and of the world our experience obliges us to acknowledge, and we are confronted all the time with at least the problem in what direction, if any, this history, or any part of it, is travelling, and whether in fact it shows any overall direction or not.

From our angle, therefore, the real reproach to traditional speculative philosophy is that it may well have been nothing like speculative enough. The more possibilities we can think of, the more chance we have of escaping from the network of parochial or anthropocentric assumptions from which we inevitably begin, and the less likely are we to fall victims to any particular undetected preconception or specially plausible error. Traditional metaphysical thought can reasonably be charged with having been too unimaginative, too content with mere variations on a limited number of more or less anthropomorphic world-models. Far more room should be found within the framework of what we recognise as philosophy—which involves in any case a semi-irrational striving to gaze beyond the outermost present bounds of our knowledge—for those who seek to draw new meanings from our experience through the utmost use of exploratory and integrative imagination in literary as much as in more narrowly " philosophic " forms : e.g., in our day, writers like D. H. Lawrence, Rilke, Valery, Kafka. They are indeed the field-workers of philosophy (on the margins of our ordinary experience, where there is no question, at least as yet, of science) rather than the theorists ; but it is just in such field-work that traditional " speculative " thought has been weakest.

(16) The foregoing marks the distinction between the present approach to philosophy and metaphysics, and that of the Logical Positivists. Their dismissal of most of the traditional content of philosophic thought as literally " nonsensical " or " meaningless " is no less disregardful of the actual psychological realities than the airy rejection by some philosophers of the entire existence of the objective world. Our sense of reality in fact rejects both attitudes in precisely the same way. We are all of us quite clear that metaphysical or traditional-philosophic questions and speculations and even discussions and arguments mean something, stand for something real and significant, however dissatisfied and frustrated many of us may feel when we try to pin down in a definite way what they do mean. We may well be as critical of the past philosophic use of language as the Logical Positivists themselves. But our criticism would be not that the traditional formulations mean nothing, but that they mean too many different things. They are manifoldly ambiguous, confused, vague and fluctuating, as well as for the most part insufficiently informed.

However, it is psychologically even if not logically obvious that in every contention or statement, every piece of theorising and debate, the philosopher concerned is trying to maintain some quite specific position which forcibly presents itself to him as both clear and right. He is seeking to hold on to some experience and consequent belief which he considers to be peculiarly significant ; or else to ward off or break up an alleged other experience threatening disruption to something he is sure of, and therefore appearing to him unreal or false. To establish unambiguously and precisely what individual thinkers are really trying to do, through the medium of our unsifted and grossly defective traditional procedures and assumptions (above all about language) is often an extremely difficult task. Sometimes indeed it is an impossible one, because in fact they are endeavouring to do several things at the same time and shifting and alternating between them. But a sufficiently searching application of psycholinguistic analysis will usually serve to establish at least the range of different things within which the objective of a particular thesis or argument must fall. And once this range has been properly brought out, even Logical Positivists can safely be challenged to pronounce it non-significant. Some or all of the positions comprised within it may be obviously wrong or inadequate or unsatisfactory ; what they are certainly not is meaningless. (The critical analyses carried out by Logical Positivists themselves often enough demonstrate the same fact.)

(17) All this still leaves formally unanswered our more specific question : what place, if any, is there on our view for the *philosophic theory of knowledge* ? However, it is clear now that the answer is largely negative. We have outlined a place for philosophy as a whole, as an attempt to make sense of or interpret our experience in its entirety. And this very role eliminates any specialised " philosophic " inquiry in a particular field ; we have seen in effect that any such local inquiry, if carried out by the only reliable and fruitful method known to us, would automatically assume the character and get drawn into the context of empirical science—in this instance the empirical psychology of knowledge. That branch of psychology, indeed, together with the rest, forms in turn a part of that comprehensive picture of our knowledge which, in conjunction with the remainder of our experience, constitutes the subject-matter for our endeavours at total integration and interpretation. But in principle it has no different *status* from the rest, and in the long run philosophy is the contemplation of the whole, or it is nothing.

Nevertheless when we have said this, we have not quite said the last word. If we look a little more nearly at the nature of our philosophic material and our philosophic problem, we shall find that in the very process of seeking to integrate its different orders of data, philosophy is inevitably led to pay a certain amount of special attention to the psychology of knowledge, because of the key position which this occupies. It can only take note of what the empirical science has actually established, and of the problems which are left, but in both aspects the psychology of knowledge is of crucial interest and importance for the philosopher's task. To bring this out explicitly, is accordingly the final object of the present essay. It will be seen that though the philosophic theory of knowledge, in the sense of the special branch of inquiry to which all cognitive problems are assigned, must disappear, the question of the relationship of knowledge to reality remains at the heart of the whole quest for an integral interpretation of our experience. Only, this quest cannot profitably commence until the empirical psychology of cognition has provided its fullest picture of all that we already know on its subject : that is the thesis with which we must end as we began.

(18) If, then, we turn to a final closer survey of the structure and materials of the philosopher's domain, as we are envisaging it here, we can say that there are four great categories of data with which he is mainly concerned.

(1) He has to take as his starting-point the latest broad scientific picture of our world ; and of course not only the most generalised physico-chemical one, but the concrete panorama of all the sciences including geology as much as astronomy, biology as much as chemistry, and empirical psychology as much as biology. This picture thus has to include (*a*) a comprehensive cross-sectional view (*b*) an equally comprehensive historical one (*c*) human beings in their double place as (i) a minutely small group of objects playing their ephemerally brief part in the objective spatio-temporal order, but also (ii) as the sole experients and knowers of the whole picture.

(2) He has to pay particular attention to unsolved problems, acknowledged question marks, anomalies, and (so far) unrelated or unintegrated facts, either within the recognised fields of the empirical sciences, or in the relations between them. For these are points from which revisions and reconstructions of as yet unknown scope in the current scientific world-picture may have to proceed.

(3) He has equally to pay particular attention to everything in human experience (familiar to him from his own case, from observation of and communion with his fellows, and from the great range of communications and self-expressions available to all of us in literature, art, etc.) which does not form part of any science, either because it is too elusive and fugitive, or because it has not so far been worked up into a systematic and tested body of knowledge or science.

(4) Finally, he cannot but take into the fullest account, as the most basic datum of all for him, his own unique individual experience-history. The features which this *shares* with other human experience-histories (to a large extent with all, and in further measure with particular groups) will form part of an *adequate* psychology. But over and above this, there is always, in the first

place, much in the individual story of each of us which is incurably singular and personal, and can neither be otherwise seized, nor just left out of account. And secondly, and more fundamentally, the philosopher's own experience-history must always remain for him something far more primary than anything else, because in the last resort it constitutes all that he himself directly has and knows.

We cannot here comment in further detail on these four classes of data. To state them is quite enough to show what a tall order of inquiry, a chimerically tall order, philosophy involves. Yet no one who seriously considers its aims can evade the conclusion that if it really seeks some sort of adequate total view or interpretation of our experience-world, however speculative, the foregoing represents the minimum range of material to which it must pay regard. If the philosopher does not do so, or cannot, so much the worse for the chances of truth or of value of his speculations. It follows of course that on the one hand he needs far more intellectual enterprise and exploratory interest in every aspect of human experience than many of his vocation have in the past displayed. On the other hand he requires vastly more help than he has hitherto received from specialised scientists in securing that minimal comprehensive picture or map of current scientific knowledge (i.e., of the whole range and burden of our most securely established truth) which is to serve as his first starting-point. The philosopher obviously cannot study all the sciences himself, or even the least one of them more than superficially : he must depend on scientists discharging one of their major duties to the community (including their own more remote co-workers) by providing at frequent intervals intelligible broad accounts of where each science has got to, for the benefit of everyone who takes a civilised interest in his human heritage. This duty is fortunately becoming more and more widely recognised and carried out ; though there is room for far more than is yet being done.

(19) However, that is by the way. What is more germane to our present approach is the rest of the philosopher's task. For (2) he is obviously also dependent in the first place on such reports as scientists can be induced to give from time to time to those members of the public who attach value to some understanding of the main unsolved problems and outstanding challenges and possible turning-points of the different sciences. But it must be confessed that whilst general accounts of the unsettled difficulties and open questions *within* individual scientific fields are not

lacking, the problems which arise out of the *relations* of some of the sciences to one another are not so well served. They are apt to appear as no *particular* scientist's business, and therefore to devolve of necessity on the philosopher. Yet in fact only scientists who together (if not separately) command the necessary competence in both or all the domains concerned, are qualified to cope with any anomalies or difficulties issuing from their mutual relations. And furthermore it is at least as important from the point of view of the integrity and growth of science itself that groups or teams of scientists should inquire into any such larger anomalies, as that they should follow up any mere local ones within each field. The inquiry, moreover, can only be carried out by those methods of factual investigation, under factual control, on which the reliability and fertility of all our scientific knowledge depends.

Meanwhile it remains true that the philosopher cannot get very much of the scientific help he needs when he comes to any problems arising out of the relations of different sciences or branches of science to one another. And far away the most difficult and perplexing and important of these questions of relationship and integration is that presented by psychology. Here indeed all his problems meet. Leaving the subject of integration for the moment, we may note that as regards our categories (3) and (4), it is only an adequate psychology which can provide him with a *comparative measure* of the data-material which he has *not* so far brought into account. What has hitherto been worked up into systematic, tested knowledge (or science) in human experience generally, and in the philosopher's in particular, forms a part of the science of psychology. What, within our experience, has not so far been incorporated in this science must however also be taken into proper consideration in the philosopher's total view. (Some of it may eventually turn out to be a key to new orders of systematic exploration and science ; but that has still to be established.)

All this is quite in line again with traditional assumptions and procedures ; the points of difference are only these : (i) On our view a large part of such additional material is merely waiting to be absorbed and integrated into our psychology, as soon as this frees itself from all its remaining philosophic shackles, and becomes truly contextual, functional and historical. (ii) What is left over is by hypothesis not yet ripe, and perhaps in part never destined to be ripe, for systematic tested knowledge; it is—whether merely so far, or permanently—too fluid, too elusive, too personal and incommunicable. Therefore it can only be taken into account very marginally, by the side of all the picture of our established or scientific knowledge. It can solely serve to reinforce, perhaps in a more concrete and living way, the other warnings which are from time to time furnished to us not to take our *current* scientific picture too literally and absolutely (the warning of the past progressive history of our scientific learning, and of all the possibilities of new discoveries still undreamt of ; the warning of the unsolved problems, the anomalies and difficulties within our scientific picture, etc.).

This attitude is clearly worlds removed from that of all those philosophers who oppose to the field of our scientific knowledge large realms of other experience, which they treat as in fact *fields of knowledge in their own right*. From these realms they thereupon draw truths, or supposed truths, that override those of " mere " science and are thought to provide the real clue to the sense or meaning of our experience as a whole. For us such an attitude is quite incompatible with any real grasp of what scientific method is or does and how it is related to all our other cognitive fumblings and gropings, naïve assumptions and muddles, errors and deadlocks. It is a view which is only possible for those who are both devoid of any psychology of knowledge and unconscious that there can be such a thing and that they lack it. But this is a position which has already been abundantly affirmed, explained and supported in all the earlier sections of the present essay.

(20) What we must return to is the special issue of the relationship of our psychological picture to the rest of our scientific knowledge. The fact is that, quite apart from local question marks, discrepant phenomena, anomalies, etc., the partial contributions offered by all the separate sciences cannot by any means be made to fuse into a single, integral total picture. Psychology, though it brings the difficulties to a head, is very possibly not their only source. The physical sciences no doubt do amalgamate readily, at least up to a point, but it does not appear certain yet that the biological ones can be joined to them without a gap, and even if this can be done, it would seem as if, at their most advanced evolutionary level, an awkward problem emerges as between the physiology of the nervous system with *its* analysis of our world, and physics and chemistry, with *their* analysis of our world. That is only secondary, however, by comparison with the apparent break, or large hiatus, between all the other sciences and psychology. That is, if the latter is the genuine thing, concerned with

complete psychic histories and only with such histories, not the too familiar hotchpotch of physiology and a limited number of psychological fragments attached to the more superficial physiological facts.

In method, we have emphasised, psychology must be at one with the other sciences, and must be built up by exactly the same processes of learning of the characteristics, groupings, and connections of its field of fact, under the direct control of that field (in the shape of the pursuit of the appropriate primary experiences, and tests of the beliefs formed from these by searching confrontation with further ones). But the outcome of that method is a comprehensive picture of a series of separate *experience*-histories in which all the other sciences themselves appear as products, and which thus in a sense embrace them and all their (experientially learnt) contents. On the other side, however, those experience-histories present themselves as only one limited aspect of organic human individuals who on the physical scientific canvas appear as no more than a vanishingly small class of objects occupying but a minute and ephemeral place in their world.

There is not necessarily any contradiction between these two separate pictures ; each when fully developed regenerates the other. Yet to integrate both of them into a single whole is quite another matter, and since it is difficult to see what more empirical science can do about it, there would seem to be room left here for almost unlimited philosophic speculation about the right integrative view. And for that purpose practically anything in our experience that is not yet science, or that baffles science, or that is too elusive or singular to become science, might, at least suggestively, be drawn in. We have very strong reasons indeed to take the physical picture as representing the underlying truth, and the psychological one as only the oddest excrescence from it, even though it is the excrescence which gives rise to the physical picture itself, as a picture. But it would be extremely rash and foolish to be dogmatic about this, so long as the excrescence is such a very odd one, and its mirroring or reproducing or (conceivably) generating relation to the rest of the physical picture so much odder still. It is not even possible, as we have already suggested, to exclude entirely the hypothesis that our whole " real " world might only be a collective human dream—or perhaps my single individual one. It would no doubt be an extraordinarily coherent and consistent performance in comparison with most of our familiar dream-experiences. But after all, these vary greatly from one another in their degrees of coherence and consistency. Therefore why should there not be something that happens to represent a more than usual degree of these qualities but is otherwise of a similar nature—and is equally a state from which we shall sometime awake (or even not awake)? In fact it is not even as tremendously consistent and coherent as all that, as we have seen. And if anyone still wishes to insist that it is too much so to be compared to a dream, let him substitute for this hypothesis that of a fixed delusional system ; those of madmen are consistent and coherent enough, and manage to turn the whole of our ordinary world into their likeness.

We may reiterate that we can do nothing with this terrifying hypothesis beyond acknowledging its conceivability. But at any rate it should keep our total world-picture philosophically open, as something that is certainly not yet self-explanatory or self-contained. The only remedy in fact against any one too fixed and rigid view is the speculative exploration of all the alternative possibilities we can think of.

(21) The philosopher, therefore, as we have seen, has grounds for paying special attention to the seam, or lack of seam, between psychology and the physical sciences. And the element of disjunction and even antithesis comes out most clearly when we focus on the psychology of knowledge (and precisely in the most adequate and comprehensive form of this), for confrontation with the physical sciences. The elements within our actual human or individual experience which have not as yet been turned even into psychology (i.e., the science which is appropriate to them, *if nothing else is*) add their own further marginal doubts and queries to the picture. Our final unique sense of our own experience-history as in the last resort all we really possess and know is of course the crux of our problem. And there are further grounds for open-mindedness, however fully we may accept the objective validity of our normal scientific world-view, as far as it (as yet) goes. We have already indicated that the very fact of knowledge is one that does not fit very easily or symmetrically into our physical scheme, and the philosopher must give due weight to this. Over and above that, however, there are all the various claimed sources of knowledge which so far remain outside our main scientific pattern of our world, and of which some may well have made out at least a prima facie case for further consideration. It may be that when they are fully investigated, they can be integrated into the same picture with the rest, perhaps by

complete assimilation, perhaps through various extensions of the picture itself. That is a matter for local scientific inquiry, not for philosophical forestalment. (We have seen that if the problem is examined by the right fact-controlled methods, that examination *is eo ipso* scientific inquiry, not philosophic speculation.) But meanwhile they have the status of possibilities, and such as *might* be of a particularly pregnant and transforming kind. In that capacity philosophic speculation must at any rate acknowledge their existence ; and it is in no worse position here than it is all round. For its equivocal essence is at all times that of an endeavour to jump ahead of our actual knowledge, or outside it, and anomalies are not only among the facts it can least afford to neglect, but may provide some of its most suggestive jumping-off boards for imaginative speculation. (This must, however, beware of merely retracing some of our traditional blind alleys, and should obviously aim at a far wider scope and secure at least some independent support from the rest of experiential evidence.)

Thus we can conclude that philosophers have strong grounds for a very special interest, not only in psychology in general but above all in the psychology of knowledge ; and in some ways most specifically in the latter's unsolved queries and problems and their possible bearings on the fundamental issues of the relation of our experience to the experienced world, and of the final status of our individual experience-history as such. In other words, whilst there is no room for a philosophic theory of knowledge as either a substitute for or a positive supplement to an adequate psychology of knowledge, philosophy as an endeavour to interpret our *total* experience-world will rightly give particular attention to the findings of such a psychology. But it must begin by *acknowledging* everything in this which has the status of established " scientific " information. And its own tentative explorations and excursions can only set out from the platform of this and the rest of our scientific knowledge as always representing what is most solid and assured within our experience as a whole.

ANALYTICAL SUMMARY

CHAPTER I—INADEQUATE PSYCHOLOGICAL DATA OF THE CURRENT PHILOSOPHIC THEORY OF KNOWLEDGE

(1) Adequate philosophic data must rest on an *adequate* description of our cognitive experience, in the context of our total experience. But traditional philosophic data represent only a narrow and defective selection.

(2) and (3) Logical analysts and positivists have shown the defects of traditional philosophic ideas, but cannot remedy them because *adequate ideas depend on adequate factual knowledge*. And all philosophers regard the " problems of knowledge " as outside the scope of factual psychology.

(4) This view is accepted by most " scientific " psychologists and strengthened by their tendency to focus on the psycho-physiological periphery. Nevertheless the recent trend has been towards a more integral approach : Gestalt view ; child psychology ; psycho-analysis ; work of Dewey and his School. Also the neglected work of J.M. Baldwin.

(5) Sketch of an answer to the formal anti-psychological case of philosophers :

  (i) the notions and assumptions of current epistemology are also empirical psychology, but they are archaic, faulty and merely sealed off from empirical correction,

  (ii) a more adequate empirical description needs no special epistemological assumptions—in fact nothing beyond our own states,

  (iii) our claim is not to supersede philosophic consideration, but only to provide authentic and stable subject-matter for this.

CHAPTER II—CHIEF FLAWS OF THE TRADITIONAL PHILOSOPHIC APPROACH. GENERAL FEATURES OF AN ADEQUATE PSYCHOLOGY OF KNOWLEDGE

(1) Psychological critique of traditional philosophers' psychology :

  (i) It still resorts to pseudo-entities like " *the* knower," " *the* mind," " *the* subject," " *the* object," Sense, Reason, Thought, etc.

  (ii) It depends on vague, questionable and often invalid data. (The difficulties in such assumed " notions " as those of " sensations," " ideas," " propositions " and " judgments.")

  (iii) Its data are severed from their context and connections.

  (iv) It restricts its attention to a narrow selection of fragments, with omission of

    (*a*) the whole *psychological* category of action,

(b) the temporal and historical character of all our experience. Action is treated as only a bodily category instead of as a distinctive mode of *experience*. Psychological elements are isolated as static entities instead of seen as parts of a single cumulative *experience-history*.

(v) It lacks the essential empirical-psychological preface to language (to allow word-meanings to be always dealt with first and apart).

(2) Positive counterpart to the above critique : the empirical psychology of knowledge must form an integral part of general psychology, which must not only be dynamic and causal, like every other empirical science, but also contextual and functional, historical and genetic.

(3) The " outside world " is only assumed in so far as validated : there is no feature of it which is not *also* an element in our psychic history, and the whole sequence of our interactions with it can be told as a history of alternation and interaction of experiences.

CHAPTER III—EXPERIENTIAL BASIS FOR THE DISTINCTION BETWEEN TRUTH AND FALSITY. THE DYNAMICS OF EXPANDING KNOWLEDGE AND GROWING LOGIC

(I) *Some Basic Working Distinctions within our Experience*

(1) The main *qualitative* groupings which we must recognise as present from the early stages of each experience-history are :
  (i) affective-conative experiences
  (ii) receptive-perceptual
  (iii) active (attentional, locomotive, operative)
  (iv) cognitive (recognitive, anticipative, representative).

(2) The distinctive features of cognitive experiences : in contrast to the above *primary* modes, they are *derivative and secondary* (re-experiencing). Receptive-perceptual experiences are not necessarily cognitive to begin with, but become so through relation to the secondary modes.

(3) The cohesiveness of our experiences in clusters and patterns.

(II) *Primary Experiential Basis for the Distinction Between Truth and Falsity*

(4) The key situation is that of recognition, with anticipation or expectation. Its first and very early form is that of : (a) recognition of a primary *experience-element* as like a previous one (b) revival of the rest of the pattern and (c) anticipation of this as about to recur in *primary* form.

(5) The crucial fact is that though mostly the new primary experience which does come fits in with expectation, sometimes it collides with this and displaces it.

(6) The relation between *expectations* of primary experiences and *actual* ones is the first and controlling basis for our distinction between truth and falsity or error.

(7) This is an authentic relation of correspondence and non-correspondence, but free from philosophic difficulties because it falls wholly within experience. Yet it is also, through its temporal character, always transcendent (to experience and belief *up to now*).

(III) *Dynamics of Expanding Knowledge and Growing Logic*

(8) The foregoing points to the main movement of our cognitive history from infancy to adulthood : the endless formation, expansion and correction of expectation-schemes on all scales ; their progressive organisation ; and their gradual transformation into representation-schemes. Perceptual experiences are the main primary mode, standing for objective actuality which expectations must conform to and are judged by.

(9) Significant features and consequences of falsified expectations :

(i) They arise from the natural course of expectation-formation and expansion.

(ii) They usually carry some degree of jar and discomfiture.

(iii) They often involve actual hurt, danger or frustration.

(iv) Thus they act as strong stimuli towards immediate readjustment and future avoidance.

(v) Their variety provides a wide range of learning opportunities lighting up in turn every factor in the situation.

(vi) The basic factors so lit up are : (*a*) the evoking stimulus (*b*) the actual further experience-contents expected. Hence the divergent possibilities of error :

(*a*) in class-*recognition* (based on the formation of cohesive class-patterns)

(*b*) in generalised belief (*about* a *correctly recognised* class).

(vii) The effects of the latter type of error :

(*a*) inhibition of expectation

(*b*) attempt at discrimination or dichotomy.

(viii) The natural development from such situations of a more and more conscious logic.

(ix) Our enduring testimony to their crucial significance :

(*a*) The recognitive-predicative structure is retained throughout the growth of empirical scientific knowledge ; and the unequivocal identifiability of the *presence* of a given object of inquiry remains all-important.

(*b*) This condition is the basis of the principle of fact-control on which all empirical science rests—only when the *presence* of the subject of a theorem or hypothesis is verified, can the truth of the latter be *tested*.

(*c*) The habit of testing confirms the need for this and leads to scientists seeking to get beliefs right by trying everything possible to prove them wrong.

G*

(*d*) Our most searching scientific tests deliberately reproduce the primary situation : expectations expressly formed (as predictions or deductions) in order to be compared with findings.

(*e*) The foregoing answers supposed difficulties about any " image " theory of thought : whether scientific representations are called images or not, they *can* be so formulated in advance as to be comparable point by point with actual findings.

(10) Acknowledgment of some over-simplifications in the above sketch :

(i) Besides the sharp antithesis of correspondence and non-correspondence, there are all degrees of partial non-correspondence (some so habitual as to be always allowed for).

(ii) There are challenging *mixtures* of correspondence and non-correspondence, to be dealt with later.

(iii) There is a large class of unexpected as distinct from anti-expected findings—but with an important functional overlap.

(11) Further empirical research is required to fill in the precise stages of some of our major cognitive advances.

(IV) *Supplementary Note about the Terms " Knowing," " Knowledge " and " Cognition "*

(12) Need for a key to the welter of confusions round these terms. Chief elements of the meaning of " knowing " :

(1) To be able to recognise
(i) experiences,
(ii) members of classes of objects, etc.

(2) To possess information.

(3) To believe with assurance, on adequate grounds, and rightly.

(4) To confront in direct apprehension.

(13), (1) (i) is the basic cognitive fact, whilst (ii) rests on our prior learning history.

(2) covers the whole content of what we normally call knowledge. Information is usually thought of as *about* some subject ; but the latter itself is represented in terms of a *complex of learnt information* (mostly recognitive).

(2) is based on the contrast with *ignorance* and always includes an admixture of error, but (*3*) rests on the contrast with *false beliefs* or mere beliefs, and so seeks formally to exclude error.

(14), (4) is the central mystery of the philosophic theory of knowledge. Our present psychological approach postpones this mystery and does not draw on sense (4), but uses the minimal subjective term " experiencing " without any advance epistemological claim. Experiencing provides the basic raw material from which beliefs and eventually knowledge emerge. The latter term is based here essentially on meaning (2), but does not exclude the *possibility* of knowing in sense (4), though enabling us to show how far we can go without this.

CHAPTER IV—EXPERIENTIAL BASIS FOR OUR BELIEF IN THE OBJECTIVE WORLD (1)

(I) *General Survey of the Problem*

(1) to (3) What the " learnt facts " about our perceptual experience have to tell us.—Philosophic criticisms are commonly disregarded, as not really *relevant* to the beliefs by which we live.

(4) to (7) The real limitations of those beliefs : common sense versus the scientific world-picture. Our naïve assumption that perception is veridical suffers the double impact of :

   (*A*) various non-veridical types of experience (optical and other illusions, etc.), and

   (*B*) the growth of the scientific world-picture. We loosely combine the latter with belief in a perceived objective world, in spite of their disparities. But there is in fact :

      (*a*) actual continuity between them and

      (*b*) the common factor of the retained status of perception as :

         (i) the chief first source of beliefs
         (ii) their activating stimulus
         (iii) above all, the final test of truth and falsity.

(8) and (9) Our belief in the objective world is not merely about actual or possible perceptual experience, but is a belief about real existences and occurrences, present, past and future. Its intimate connection with the notion of causal control.

(10) The threefold way in which our objective world-picture is built up from :
   (i) discrete objects
   (ii) their framework or setting
   (iii) the order of events.
   The sustained status and importance of objects.

(II) *Preliminary Cross-Sectional Approach to Common Sense Adult Belief*

(11) An analysis of our state on waking up any morning : the perceptual component and its characters and attributes.

(12) and (13) What we believe about this component and on what good grounds. The way in which the most diverse types of experiences *converge* in our conviction of an order of things which is objectively there :
   (i) to be perceived
   (ii) to be encountered in reciprocal action
   (iii) to be learnt about
   (iv) to be increasingly and more and more *correctly* known.

(14) and (15) The part played in this scheme and its development by

(i) our own (perceived) body

(ii) other human beings

(iii) larger cycles of planned actions and relations, and

(iv) our common share of errors and failures.

Summary of the main features of our experience as integrated in our acknowledgment of the objective world. The whole scheme is constantly re-tested and re-confirmed by every character and aspect of our *further* experience.

CHAPTER V—EXPERIENTIAL BASIS FOR OUR BELIEF IN THE OBJECTIVE WORLD (2)

(I) *Genetic Approach : a Preliminary Difficulty*

(1) to (4) We depend on " behaviouristic " evidence for the reconstruction of our early psychic life, but in spite of various complications we have very good grounds for admitting it. Its *progression* is a chief key to our picture of early experience. The traditional philosophic assumptions about this are mainly gratuitous. The minimal pattern of our early primary experiencing is, once more, affective-conative, perceptual and active.

(5) The importance of ensuring that the *psychological* story is complete. We have to show how the child comes by the very notion of the physical world ; of his own existence ; of his interaction with the physical world ; of his position in it ; and of his own picture of it. Behaviouristic evidence is chiefly a source of genetic cues and warnings ; our cross-sectional analysis is a check and touchstone.

(II) *The Chief Types and Phases of Early Experience which Go to Build Up our World-Picture*

(6) How attentional objects first emerge in the attentional field. The effect of our ability to *maintain, relinquish, recover* and *extend* particular experience-contents. The effect of our characteristic experienced *field.*

(7) How attentional objects in the attentional field develop into " real " objects in a " real " field. The case of moving foci which visual attention *follows.* The effect of multiple foci and their shifting relations in a continuing field.

(8) The contributions of tactile experience and attention ; of auditory and olfactory happenings ; and of the child's experience of his own bodily movements, of being moved and of locomotion. The growth of more and more forms of operative experience : activities (*a*) upon objects (*b*) with objects and (*c*) with some upon others.

(9) The integration of the child's own body into his given spatial field and among its objects. Whilst sharing practically all features with these, it combines this fact with a unique relation to the child's whole experience. Our growing tendency to equate psychological objectiveness with existence in space outside our own body.

(10) How the order of " real " *occurrences* develops concomitantly with that of " real " *objects* within a single objective world. The significance of changes *within* the perceptual field whilst our attention remains fixed. Our perception of changes versus changes in our perception. Complexities of the distinction, which nevertheless develops into the far-reaching one between " real " and " merely subjective " happenings. The objective past and history versus our personal past and history (including perceptual).

(11) The building up of our normal picture of a spatio-temporal world with diverse occupants and occurrences, and a comprehensive geography and history. Our progressive discovery of multitudes of partly similar, partly different objects and events. Our marshalling of diverse types of objective entities, substances, qualities, states, parts, groupings, situations, occasions, processes, cycles, etc. The development of recognition, anticipation and planned action. " Facts " ; true knowledge ; errors and their correction ; our gaps of ignorance and their filling in.

(12) The fundamental contributions of our acknowledgment, among objects, of the class of human ones. The child (*a*) becomes aware of all the similarities to himself of these objects (*b*) sees nevertheless that they are continuous with others less and less like them (*c*) discovers more and more that they pass through experience-courses *parallel* to his own and *interchangeable* with them, but going beyond them, so that he can always draw on their wider range. Thus at length he learns to acknowledge and participate in the general human pool of experience and knowledge.

(13) All these discoveries depend on our *acknowledgment* of the objective world, which is, however, in turn *confirmed and immensely enlarged* by them. The information which the child obtains from others is no mere hearsay, but

    (*a*) fits into the groundwork of his direct experience

    (*b*) gets translated into endless further beliefs and expectations which are sooner or later tested and mostly confirmed. (But it is true that this very fact creates room for a considerable admixture of undetected or uncorrected error.)

(14) Retrospect : the main progressive stages of belief in an objective world pass continuously into one another. Each *builds on those before*, is *in turn verified*, and so allows *further building*. Hence the endless *cumulative* addition of substance and depth to the child's scheme of beliefs, both in actual content and in verification.

(15) and (16) A partial qualification arises from the very facts of the controlling relationship of perceptual experience to affective-conative, leading to the acknowledged dependence of the latter on the objective world. The primary controlling object on which all the child's early life turns is a personal one, viz. his mother ; who is soon joined by other personal powers. The resulting early world-picture is one of spontaneous and incalculable powers, which use other objects as instruments, and are open to influence (but not control) by bare expressions of needs and wishes, by appeal and invocation, and sometimes apparently by feeling as such. These " powers " are progressively assimilated to other objects, but in most communities the end-picture is still of a limited learnable object-order subject to a vague penumbra of overriding personal powers. Only in our society has the learnable object-order been expanded into a vast (tested and verified) non-personal world-scheme.

(17) Any strictly genetic account of the child's cognitive history should start from the central cycle of his mainly affective interchanges with his mother, and marshal the rest of the story round this, but the same pattern would emerge. The original cycle shrinks successively as the ambit of experience enlarges, whilst concurrently the nucleus of immediate *perception* shrinks within an expanding system of *beliefs*. But the paramountcy of perception as source and test of beliefs is maintained even as its *occurrence* becomes more and more contingent. Knowledge is the reflection of what *is so, whether we happen to know of it or not.*

(18) The most fundamental dividing line in our experience is not that between our total *perceptual material* and the rest, but between our whole history up to a given moment, and any new perceptual experience then supervening. The latter continually tests at different points and in different ways the system of beliefs shaped from the former. But this is chiefly made up from past " new " perceptual material and most of it satisfies all our tests, our earlier failures having merely served to strengthen the system. Our fully verified beliefs pass indeed by insensible gradations into theories, conjectures and mere imaginings, but despite borderline uncertainties and aberrations, we have no difficulty by and large in maintaining our division between fantasy and fact.

(19) Note about the margins and limits of our structure of cumulatively verified beliefs :

(i) We have deceptive experiences like mirror images, optical illusions, dreams, delusions, etc. Most of these are just orders of falsified expectations which lead to the segregation of special expectation-systems that fit satisfactorily into our main structure. On the other hand habitual proneness to hallucinations and delusion is recognised as a breakdown of the reality-sense and of the capacity for independent life.

(ii) Nevertheless there can be no ultimate certainty about what is always only a reading of our experience *so far*. Hallucinations and dreams exemplify the possibility of total error ; though even so we should have to maintain all our habitual distinctions and beliefs *within* our system of error, because our continuing experience demands and confirms them.

(20), (iii) Our stress on perceptual experience neither excludes nor prejudges the claims of other possible sources of knowledge. Among many historical claimants, some accept the common sense world and invoke evidence within this, some set up rival and superior realms of reality. Further comment is postponed till our last chapter but

    (*a*) all claims must take into account the immense scope and strength of our established perception-based knowledge, which we cannot escape

    (*b*) claims which affirm non-perceptual reality must specify what they *mean* by this and by what criteria it can be *distinguished* from " mere " feeling or thinking. *Through use of the same symbols*, we are led to transfer claims and titles hinging on perceptual experience to other meanings or definitions with no least right to them.

CHAPTER VI—EXPERIENTIAL BASIS FOR OUR BELIEF IN CAUSALITY

(1) and (2) Our common sense notion of causality and its confusions. What is necessary is to assemble and integrate all the experience-elements separately represented in it.

(3) The shortcomings of our pseudo-scientific notion of invariable succession. What we have to take account of are all the child's experiences of :

    (*a*) his control by objects

    (*b*) his counter-control of objects

    (*c*) his observations of the control of objects by one another

    (*d*) his observations of the linkages of successive happenings with one another, and the occasional failures of these linkages

    (*e*) and (*f*) his ability to seek and find *key* happenings which control any given happenings.

(4), (*a*) Control of the child by objects is experienced as :

    (i) control of his attentional activity and passivity

    (ii) control of his states of satisfaction and non-satisfaction.

  (*b*) Counter-control of objects by the child is experienced through :

    (i) his effect-producing energising and play

    (ii) all his progressive activities upon objects, in order to influence and control his own feeling states through them.

  (*c*) The child concurrently *notes* all round him an endless variety of actions of objects on objects, and their outcomes. And these in turn fit in with (*a*) and (*b*), and support and extend them.

(5) and (6) (*d*) At the same time he is continually watching sequences of events, forming expectations, correcting these, and linking *intrusive happenings* with *previous intrusive ones* found to serve as keys and instruments of control.

(*e*) and (*f*) The foregoing leads to the explicit causal questions : " What makes . . . ? " " What made . . . ? " Also to a variety of other causal question-forms, including the search for motives and purposes. And suitable inquiry leads regularly to the discovery of a verifiable answer.

(7) An integrated account of our common sense causal notion and its component experiences :

    (i) The *active or operative core* is, most typically, the introduction of a new agency or factor into a given field (or the alteration or increase of an existing one).

    (ii) There is always a *qualifying and limiting penumbra*, in the shape of a hierarchy of co-controlling factors, preparatory, predisposing and permissive conditions, etc.

    (iii) *Interfering, deflecting or preventing* " *causes* " bring back under the causal rule cases where it had appeared to break down.

(8), (iv) *Reciprocal action of* " *cause* " *and* " *effect* " :— If a particular agency or specific event is envisaged as " *the* " cause, no attention is usually paid to the counter-effect produced on it. But on a more adequate view, a reaction of the field on the agent, or a cumulative interaction, is the rule.

    (v) *Negative causality*. The cessation or removal of previously operative agencies often first makes us aware of their previous participation.

    (vi) *Static or passive causality—dependence and interdependence*. Breakdowns of apparent causal rules bring to light factors on which the production of the effect *also* depends. In general not only changes but equally the maintenance of given states of affairs is found to depend on the continuance of particular factors and conditions. A further advance is to the notion of schemes of *inter*dependences within a given system, controlling either its stability, or its return to this after disturbance.

(9), (vii) *Distinction between functional-structural and historical causality*. On the one hand we have knowledge of *classes* of things within which learning is transferable, on the other we have specific knowledge of *individual things*, situations, etc. Outstanding cases of the latter type are individual autobiography and world-history.

(10) Our resulting double form of causal inquiry :

    (i) What causes events of *class* A to happen ?

    (ii) What caused a *specific event* ' A ' to happen here and now ?

The former leads to the functional-structural knowledge of most of our sciences ; the latter to the historical knowledge of geology, evolutionary biology, etc. Psychology is a special case, seeking class-knowledge, but class-knowledge of individual cumulative histories. Our object here is to study typical history-patterns and typical variations, in relation to variations of endowment and setting.

(11) Retrospect and conclusion : we have a vast body of experiences which account for every aspect and component of our common sense belief in causality. Yet this remains muddled, and commonly substitutes some fragment (varying widely according to person and occasion) for the full picture. However, on a systematic approach the latter tends to emerge, and the very gamut of our confusions testifies to it. But (*a*) causal questions are sometimes carried beyond any meaning, and (*b*) we fall into special muddles and overlaps with the notion of explanation. This is quite distinct and must be separately examined.

CHAPTER VII—THE PSYCHOLOGY OF PUZZLEMENT AND OF EXPLANATION

(1) Our notion of explanation is the completion of the story of *how* we learn from experience.

(2) and (3) The distinction between our ideas of causality and of explanation : the former stands for a characteristic of the objective world ; the latter for information capable of a particular cognitive function. " Explanation " is typically new or additional information which relieves puzzlement and resolves a cognitive clash.

(4) and (5) " Why " questions and their many meanings. The primary one is that of inquiry about motives and purposes, which the child finds to be an invaluable key, and applies universally till he learns its limitations. But by his 4th/5th year he discovers a distinct second sense : the quest for relief and help in *any* experience of anti-expectedness and unexpectedness.

(6), (i) Other meanings which branch out from the same root :

(*a*) general mode of inquiry about causes

(*b*) inquiry about logical reasons or grounds (for assertions or propositions)

(*c*) affective meanings : surprise, protest, vexation, etc.

(ii) We must take care to distinguish between questions which seek particular types of *predefined* information, and the one large group of " why " questions which seek an unknown X capable of functioning as explanation. The former are recognised keys to growing bodies of information (What is ? What makes ? Of what is . . . made ? Where ? How ? etc. Also " Why ? " in its several specific information-seeking senses). The explanation-seeking " why " comes later and particularly expresses *ignorance of what the right kind of information might be*. The picture is somewhat blurred because our growing experience of explanations received leads to " why's " which seek now familiar types ; but the open " why " always survives.

(7) We have a wide range of alternative ways of resolving puzzlement in cases of open " why's," from the mere discovery of misperception to the far-reaching reconstruction of some previous scheme of belief. In between fall various types of uncovery of unconsidered factors—qualifying circumstances, intervening causes, missing links, etc. And also the great class of pseudo-explanations : by " ideas," verbal paraphrases, reified abstractions, etc. Explanations must be *both* capable of explaining *if* true, *and* true. Our accepted standard of explanation is the key either to the premature closure or to the unlimited advance of our learning processes.

(8) The epistemic " why " question thus marks the parting of the ways. Our questioning state is one of general unrest ; an accepted explanation is the return to rest. The child takes over from his parents and other adults his criteria of what constitutes a valid explanation—criteria which decide when he will be satisfied and when he will continue inquiring.—Our current criteria are in fact still very imperfect, except those implicit in actual scientific investigation. Indeed even the *theory* of scientific theories remains so far in an unsatisfactory state largely for lack of the foundation of a stable and effective theory of truth. This is provided by the present psychological account of truth and error (based on temporal correspondence), which leads directly to the functional history and operative criteria of explanation, up to the level of fullest scientific achievement.

CHAPTER VIII—THE BEARINGS OF AN ADEQUATE PSYCHOLOGY OF KNOWLEDGE ON THE PHILOSOPHIC THEORY OF KNOWLEDGE

(1) and (2) Before the place left for the philosophic theory of knowledge can be determined, there are omissions in our picture still to be considered. But these omissions must be examined against the massive structure of our cumulative learning from experience, under the aegis of the principle of fact-control, both physical and (" merely ") psychological.

(3) We must distinguish between thoughts that
   (i) make no truth-claim
   (ii) claim only psychological truth
   (iii) claim truth in the perceptual-objective field
   (iv) claim truth in any distinct further field.
There are two questions :
   (1) Have we any sources, other than those hitherto considered, of truth-claims in either the psychological or the perceptual field ?
   (2) Have we any sources of truth-claims in any other sort of field ?—And how far are any such claims established ?

(4) These again are specific problems for empirical psychology ; the second indeed calls first of all for psycho-linguistic elucidation, which must itself be empirical. Whatever else such truth-claims may involve, they are psychological phenomena to begin with and must be examined in their context, both for their own understanding and for their bearing on that context.

(5) Some of the main truth-claims which are believed to be independent of perceptual learning : Group I, wholly or chiefly directed to either the perceptual-physical or the psychological world ; Group II, professing to transcend both these worlds.

(6) GROUP I.

(i) and (ii) : *Innate (or inherited) and instinctive knowledge.* There are widespread and striking examples of the latter (if not of the former) in the animal world ; it may well be present also in human beings, but is clearly limited in scope and heavily overlaid with learnt information. In any case it is very fallible.

(iii) " *Intuitive* " *knowledge.* This is largely discredited ; very often it is no more than swift implicit inference, and frequently plain error. Any authentic residuum needs demonstration by searching empirical inquiry.

(7), (iv) *Logical inference.* This is a genuine source of unlearnt knowledge, which would seem to go much beyond the syllogistic pattern derivable from expectation situations. There are diverse forms of relational inference which call for further empirical psychological study. But

(i) it is subject to many pitfalls shown by falsified conclusions (= expectations) ;

(ii) in any case, where the related beliefs are learnt ones, the conclusion is no more reliable than both or all the premises, and often brings out latent weaknesses or limitations in them.

(v) *Logically constructed knowledge.* Chiefly the difficult case of mathematics, to be considered later.

(8), (vi) to (xi) *Prophecy ; veridical dreaming ; clairvoyance ; spirit communication ; telepathy ; occult knowledge.* These modes have usually been grouped in the past as pertaining to the " supernatural," but they mostly refer to phenomena held to occur in and to be verifiable within the perceptual-objective world. More recently it has been claimed that many of these phenomena have been scientifically established (in the case of telepathy as unlearnt knowledge in the psychological field). Most of them are still controversial and the past approach to them has been open to serious scientific criticisms ; but they are obviously all a matter for empirical *psychological* research.

(9) GROUP II.

(xii) and (xiii)   *Revelation and mystical vision.* These again raise
inescapable *psychological* questions : if fantasies or delusions can *pretend* to be revelation or mystical vision, by what
criteria do we distinguish between them and the real thing ?
(If perceptual tests are to be excluded, what others are to be
substituted ?)—Philosophic discussion of these topics is
always caught in the familiar verbal-factual slide ; the only
approach capable of definite results is the empirical psychological one (first linguistic, then psychological-factual).

(10), (xiv)-(xvi)   *Religious, ethical and aesthetic experience.* These are
often claimed to be distinctive modes of experience, which
disclose or point to distinctive orders of reality. They are
usually regarded as philosophic themes, but merely lead
into the accustomed dialectical difficulties. The first question
is again the psycho-linguistic one : just what is *meant* here
by " reality " if by hypothesis it is not perceptual-objective ?
The next question is once more the substantive one of
criteria of distinction between deceptive or erroneous claims
and authentic ones. But it is in fact an initial mistake to
take the adult forms of these experiences at their face-value ;
they are products of a long history which needs to be traced.
It may be suggested that if this were done, little of the
original problem may remain ; but in any event the full
psychological story must come first.

(11) Return to sub-group (v). *The problem of mathematics.* The latter
was originally thought of as the model of what all " science "
(including philosophical) should be ; but the attempted general
transfer of its assumptions and methods obviously broke down.
That however leaves the question of what the unique success of
mathematics itself rests upon. This needs to be approached as a
problem of cognitive psychology—but by psychologists with
adequate mathematical competence.

(12) Comments from a purely psychological angle. The current tautological view would effectively dissolve our problem, but suggests
psychological misgivings over the notion of tautology and its ordinary complete barrenness. Something more would seem to be required to account for the extraordinary fruitfulness and power of
mathematics. There are tentative pointers in certain *passive* properties of objects : their susceptibility to various operations which
can be performed without otherwise changing them—aggregation
and separation, superimposition and inclusion. Here again there
is a case for full factual-psychological investigation.

(13) What now is left for the philosophic theory of knowledge ? It
is an untenable view that psychology surveys facts and epistemology considers problems. Problems arising out of known facts
must be pursued by further factual inquiry (e.g., chemical or

geological researches are not broken off at points of difficulty and handed over to philosophers). Nor does philosophy stand for *superior methods* of dealing with problems too refractory for empirical science ; the latter on the contrary signifies a break-away from the *defects* of philosophic method.

(14) The real issue is what scope there is left for philosophy as such. It is accepted here that it represents the genuine question whether we can arrive at any comprehensive *interpretation* firstly of the sum of our empirical scientific knowledge and secondly of our experience as a whole (including such knowledge—but also elements which do not, or do not yet, form part of any science, and furthermore any *unlearnt* knowledge which we believe has been established).

(15) Such a demand may be found incapable of satisfaction, but it must be *considered* (by empirical scientific methods and canons). The enterprise is more or less comparable, on a vaster scale, with that of scientific explanatory hypotheses. The criteria for the latter, which should be equally applicable, are : illumination of what is known, uncovery of things previously unknown, and direct verifiability. But in respect of our total experience there is no hope at best of a higher status than that of speculations—which need to be as various, imaginative and bold as possible. (Note the " field " work of literary explorers of the margins of experience.)

(16) Distinction of this approach from that of the Logical Positivists : where they assert " meaninglessness," the present diagnosis is of muddles of many meanings. From this muddle it is both possible and important to sift out and marshal specific sets.

(17) Return to the question of the place left for the philosophic theory of knowledge. We are led to the largely negative answer that the role of philosophy excludes any specialised inquiry in a particular field, which, if rightly conducted, always leads to specific *science*. But nevertheless this role calls for close attention to the *psychology* of knowledge, with its key position.

(18) Philosophy is concerned with four main categories of data : (1) The broad scientific picture of our world. (2) Unsolved problems, anomalies, and unintegrated facts within the empirical sciences or in the relations between them. (3) Everything else in human experience generally which does not form part (at least so far) of any recognised science. (4) The philosopher's own unique individual experience-history.

(19) Particular difficulties under (2) arise from the relations between certain of the sciences, but need first of all the attention of teams of scientists. A special position applies in the case of psychology which, dealing with experience as such, throws into contrasted relief whatever in this has not so far been turned into science, or may be incapable of being.

(20) Furthermore psychology presents peculiar obstacles to integration with the rest of empirical science. It exhibits comprehensive experience-histories in which all sciences appear as elements and products ; but these sciences exhibit those histories themselves as only an aspect of a small and ephemeral class of local objects. Unlimited room is thus left for philosophic speculation about the right mode of integration of these two pictures. There are grounds for emphasising the physical one—but even the most opposite extreme, viz., the " dream " hypothesis, remains an open possibility.

(21) The above disjunction is thrown up most clearly in connection with the psychology of knowledge. Hence philosophers' strong grounds for interest in this. But (just as in other fields) we must begin by acknowledging everything which is or can be established as science, because that is always what is most solid and assured in our experience as a whole.

INDEX

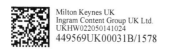

Milton Keynes UK
Ingram Content Group UK Ltd.
UKHW022050141024
449569UK00031B/1578